NEUROPLASTICITY

Newest Guide to Working Brain Plasticity

(Master Neuroplasticity for Recovery and Growth
After Stroke)

Kelly Roach

I0222730

Published By Bengion Cosalas

Kelly Roache

All Rights Reserved

*Neuroplasticity: Newest Guide to Working Brain Plasticity
(Master Neuroplasticity for Recovery and Growth After
Stroke)*

ISBN 978-1-77485-294-1

Table of Contents

Introduction

This book outlines the most effective steps and strategies on how to better understand the process of brain plasticity and how you can swiftly and effectively alter your brain's capabilities to be most effective and efficient to achieve the desired goals in your life!

Our brains are extremely amazing that most people don't ever even realize the nearly infinite possibilities that our brains can offer. We tend to let the circumstances of life to determine where our physical lives go and not realize that any change to the physical world first needs to result in a change to the mental realm.

Brain Plasticity can help you understand by advancing neuroscience how to create new neural pathways that will ensure the outcomes you want to achieve will become reality. If you're feeling like you're not getting anywhere in your life and you're starting to believe you're not able then you must make use of the brain's ability to change.

Also, you should not waste time. If you're looking to begin living your life in the way you would like start, then go through this now and begin changing your mind in the fastest way feasible.

Chapter 1: What is Neuroplasticity?

The idea of neuroplasticity has become popular in a rapid manner. It is understandable that a lot of people are discussing this concept because it's an exciting topic to consider. This is what makes the term "neuroplasty" somewhat of an "buzz term" and we need to determine exactly what it is.

Neuroplasticity is a broad term that refers to your brain's ability to adapt its functions and physically. Neuroplasticity may occur as an outcome of the environment or repetitive thoughts as well as habitual behavior and intense emotions.

The idea that brains are malleable could be traced back to the 1800's however this was just a theorized. The relatively recent development of MRI has proved that a malleable, also known as a "plastic" brain actually, a fact. Science has proved that the brain's capacity to transform is real without doubt.

Recent developments have altered the belief system that says the adult brain is stationary or is even wired during developmental times that are thought to be vital in the early years of the early years of childhood. While your brain might be more flexible during the first phases in life and even though the ability to change decreases as you the passage of time, it has been established that the process of plasticity continues throughout life for humans. Everyone can utilize the power of neuroplasticity even the elderly.

Brains can be malleable. According to TheFreeDictionary.com, malleable is defined as:

malleable:

1. It is able to be bent, shaped bent or dragged out with hammering or pressure, without breaking.

flexible, moldable, plastic, pliable, pliant, supple, workable.

2. Easy to modify or alter:

ductile, elastic, flexible, impressionable, plastic, pliable, pliant, suggestible, supple.

3. Capable of adapting to changes in the environment. Capable of adapting or being modified. The ability to be changed and adjusted in order to satisfy specific or different requirements.

adaptable, adaptive, adjustable, elastic, flexible, pliable, pliant, supple.

We are able to shape and mold our brains!

Chapter 2: Scientific Proof That

Brain Plasticity Functions at Any Age

As we get older our brains continue to undergo growth and growth. The most surprising and unexpected discoveries of our modern times is that adults too are able to increase the power of their brain by enhancing their brain's plasticity. There was an old belief in which it was believed that only children could develop by enhancing their brains. However, with the most advanced technology at hand the old idea has been proven wrong.

Neurogenesis, which is also called brain plasticity, refers to the brain's ability to change throughout the human lifespan. It happens because of the development of new connections between every brain cell. It can affect or improve the brain's function. There is evidence from science that the re-inforcing and strengthening of brain cell connectivity occurs regardless of whether a person is at an advanced age.

The evidence was drawn from various kinds of data. For instance when a study was conducted by taxi drivers in London researchers discovered that they had a higher level of brain-related plasticity as in comparison to bus drivers. The phenomena was explained as the result of bus drivers have an established route that they follow. However taxi drivers in London must be acquainted with 25 000 streets. The brain part which is associated with navigation and map reading increased as well, and this happens at all age groups. This proves that the brain has an active mechanism for neurologic growth , as opposed to the idea that it just housed thousands of neurons as they were waiting for their deaths.

In addition, it was found that there is a degree of plasticity in people who can speak an additional language other than their native language. It is believed that the acquisition of a second language can be only possible due to major changes within the internal structures of our brain. It is located in the back of the brain cell.

The majority of people who speak multiple languages have large back regions (specifically on the left) in the brain.

There were differences within the brains of those who prefer to play music, as opposed to people who aren't. The brain's volume of musicians was found to be the highest in professionals. However, those who do not play any music whatsoever have the least brain volume.

Furthermore, a large amount of abstract learning in nature can cause several significant changes in the brain. In a different study the brains of students were examined prior to and after the exam (three months between). The brains of the students were found experiencing changes within regions involved in memory and learning retrieval. The same thing did not occur to people in control groups, those who didn't do any preparation or studying for an examination. The brains of the control group did not show any changes. the brains of the people who didn't study for the examination.

These little bits of evidence promote the notion of the brain in adulthood being more flexible than we think it is. The brain grows throughout one's lifetime. Similar to that it is possible for the brain to degrade. This is possible if one is not doing something to increase his intelligence level. If you want to keep or even improve the condition that your brain is in, you must to perform physical and mental exercises. It is also essential to engage in environmental enrichment activities.

If you're now an adult, it's not too late to improve your skills by altering brain's function. There are numerous computer programs that could assist you in achieving this. Other suggestions you can try: start writing using your hand that is not your dominant one or master a language you have never heard of, listen to various birds' songs and try to determine what species of bird they are, discover an instrument you've never heard of and develop new math techniques.

Chapter 3: Overhaul Your Attitude And Shape A More Positive Mind

After reading the chapter before You now understand that due to the flexible character of the brain it has the ability to acquire new abilities. The third chapter we'll explore this further and discuss how you can adopt to increase your ability to learn. Neuroplasticity isn't just helpful in expanding the vocabulary of your children or helping them learn how to play an instrument. It also opens the door to the improvement of your abilities in your life, and a new perspective about life generally. This chapter you'll discover how the brain's ability to change is a huge advantage in making adjustments to the way you live your life.

Thinking positively is an key skill

Some individuals are born positive thinkers, and this aspect of a person's personality is fixed. While it is true that there is a genetic component to personality characteristics, there is growing evidence that if one is willing to put forth the effort to alter your thoughts the brain and actions will assist in moving towards a positive direction.

The people who have mastered their ability to think positively are likely succeed in every aspect of their lives. It is important to note that being positive doesn't mean you willfully ignore constructive criticism or are unwilling to accept the reality. Instead, it implies that you are confident in your abilities and that the majority of scenarios contain at least possibility of a positive result. Like driving around London often helps to build neurons in the taxi driver that are responsible for a successful spatial navigation, repetition of positive thinking can help you instantly look for positive outcomes when you encounter the roadblocks in life. This will ultimately help you develop resilience, which guards against depression. It also helps to overcome any challenges that life presents to you.

Depression, neuroplasticity, as well as practicing positive thoughts

Depression's effects on brain are important in helping us understand the concept of neuroplasticity and its relationship to mood and cognitive functioning. Recent research has shown that depression isn't only a state of mind and experience. It is rather a neurochemical event with many ramifications that go beyond sensation of feeling "down" and "sad." The term "depression" refers to a psychological illness characterized by a variety of emotional, psychological physical and mental symptoms, such as feelings of sadness, of hopelessness, thoughts about suicide or death and a loss of enthusiasm for previously enjoyed activities as well as changes in weight and appetite, or unrelated aches and pains without a clear physical cause and a tendency to be withdrawn from social settings.

Psychologists believe there are many underlying causes which could be the cause or contribute to depression, which include the genetic predisposition to depression as well as neurological imbalance. Certain of these could be out of your control. However there's a lot of evidence suggesting that the primary factor that keeps depression in the first place is a person's way of thinking. Simply put, those suffering from depression are prone to view the world in an unadaptive way , which keeps them trapped in a loop of negative thoughts and negative behavior, as well as withdrawing from the world surrounding them. To overcome the feelings of despair and despair that frequently befall depression and keep the depression going, it's crucial that someone suffering from depression retrains their brain to perceive the world around them in a more positive manner.

This is the basis for the concept of psychotherapy referred to by the name of Cognitive Behavioral Therapy, or CBT. The basic idea behind CBT is it's not just the events that happen to us in life that makes us feel certain ways the main factor that determines our mood is the personal meaning that we assign to events that happen outside. CBT experts believe the primary difference that separates people who suffer from depression from people who are healthy mentally is that people with depression frequently fall back to negative perceptions of the world. That is, when depression is a problem you constantly tell you that life is not a good location, that you'll suffer injuries often and that there's no reason to believe that things will improve. This kind of thinking becomes "normal," and over time, you might not be aware of how negativist mindset is ingrained.

You are aware that neurons that are firing together tend to create a network. You can think negative thoughts regularly and they'll begin to reflect your current reality. The result is noticeable in the mind. Brain scans that compare the brains of those who suffer from depression and those without discovered that mental illness may cause a state known as "negative neuroplasticity" where certain thoughts and behaviors become ingrained and persist as symptoms. The research conducted by the University of Michigan using a brain scanning procedure called positron emission tomography (PET) revealed that people who suffer from depression that are not treated have less serotonin receptors than people who were not diagnosed with the disease. This is significant since in order to be content and manage our mood our brains have to have the ability to create the proper use of the neurotransmitter.

The findings of other studies have shown that those suffering from depression tend to have shrinkage in the hippocampus. This in the end makes them susceptible to mood disorders and impaired memory functions. The more depressive episodes one suffers more severe the severity of hippocampal degeneration. Because depression is a risk factor in the progression of Alzheimer's disease and that the hippocampus can be one of the first areas of the brain to become affected in people suffering from the condition, it's likely that the primary cause of this connection is an impaired hippocampal area. Further research is required in this area, however, the main message here is that depression affects the human brain.

However, there is plenty of evidence that suggests that psychotherapy that involves ensuring that people who are suffering from depression learn new ways of looking at the world, and are challenged by their negative thoughts, is a successful treatment. If you've been suffering from depression or negative thinking for a number of years there's a reason to optimism because our brains do not stop developing, so with the correct treatment and a change in your behavior you can repair the harm.

Exercise: Refusing Negative Thinking

Though negative thoughts are commonplace in depression, the majority of us experience their negative impacts from time to time. If you let them get excessive mental space However, you may start to notice your attitudes towards other people and your life as a whole decrease. This could have a negative impact on your daily conduct. This is a routine exercise utilized in the hands of CBT therapists.

1. Find a negative idea that you are prone to thinking about often. It could be related to your situation in the social realm (e.g. "I do not have friends") or your self-image ("I'm incapable of doing anything and cannot accomplish things") or to the world at large ("Everyone is selfish and is only looking to make a profit"). Write it down and evaluate its credibility on a scale from 1 to 10 10, with 10 being the number that indicates you believe this idea as absolutely accurate.

2. It's time to go on a detective mission. Do you know any evidence to support this is indeed real? Note down the evidence you have for this idea. Then, look at it from an alternative perspective - if were to argue the opposite argument What evidence would be offered to support of the argument that this view isn't the case? For instance, if you wrote "I'm incapable of doing anything and I'm unable to accomplish anything" in Step 1, you're

now to recognize that while you might not be as skilled in a particular field as you'd like however, you've been successful in other fields and have developed other abilities.

3. After you have reviewed the evidence, consider whether you are able to accept your belief that is not true to the reality. If you've put in the effort to produce evidence that supports each side (i.e. the assertion being true or false) then you will find that its influence over you is diminished.

4. In addition consider whether or not your negative thinking could be beneficial. Even if it's accurate (which is extremely unlikely) what can you gain from reliving the thought as if it were true? Negative thought patterns rarely lead to positive changes. Think about the advantages of allowing yourself the freedom to change your thinking.

The reason this exercise works is as it makes you be aware that the world isn't just black and white, and that even the most deeply held negative thoughts aren't resistant to the influence that is critical thinking! If you practice this practice whenever you find yourself falling to negative thinking, you'll quickly learn to confront negative thoughts instead of allowing it to pass and accepting it to be a "normal situation." For the next few days take a vow to yourself that you're not going to sit and allow the unhelpful negativity that your brain is able to throw at you. Instead, commit to view negative negative thoughts as negative mental habits you can overcome by perseverance and determination.

Many people find keeping a journal can help to identify and combat negative thoughts. It's not feasible to record all negative thoughts that enters your mind however, you could benefit from your journal to note down certain themes or devising alternative solutions to negative thoughts that come up repeatedly. Journaling is much simpler to adhere to once you have made it an habit. Keep in mind that if you repeat a task repeatedly your brain will start to expect it , and you'll be uneasy if you break your routine. It is likely that you clean your teeth in the day and night without thinking about it. This is because you've done the same procedure hundreds of times in the past. It's the same in the case of journaling, or any other new habit you wish to establish. Establish a date and time to journal in the next the next 30 days. We'll return to setting goals and habit-setting in Chapter 4.

What is the reason "Fake it until you achieve it" is actually effective - the Facial Feedback Hypothesis

The old adage of "Fake it until you can achieve the mistake!" may sound trite and useless if you're feeling down However, psychologists have found that this cliche has merit. Many of us believe that our moods and body language are connected in the following way: When we experience some event or memory when a certain emotion arises within us the way we communicate alters because of it. We smile when we're content, and slump in our chairs when depressed and so on.

While this may be true but did you know that there's a lot of evidence to suggest that it can also work in the reverse direction? Smile because you're content, but if decide to smile, even if you're unhappy or down chances are you'll notice a significant improvement of your attitude. This phenomenon, in which the brain is able to receive information from the facial expression as well as other body language in that the person is able to feel their mood or change in attitude it is known as"Facial Feedback" Hypothesis.

The first studies conducted in this field included volunteers who were instructed to place the pencil in between their teeth while they watched cartoon strips. People who were required to hold an unidirectional pencil between their teeth, rated the cartoons as more enjoyable than those who were instructed to hold the pencil in a way that they did not have to make their lips smile. Researchers concluded that since the group holding the pencil horizontally was effectively induced to adopt an "happy" expression and their brains saw the cartoons as funny. Another study has revealed that taking "power postures" (such as standing with your legs separated in a straight back and fingers on the hips) can boost confidence when faced with nerve-wracking situations.

These findings are fascinating as they indicate the existence of neural pathways that enable our brains to connect particular facial expressions, gestures and postures with specific mood states. So why not make the most of these neural circuits already in place?

Practice: Test Face Feedback Yourself

The more often you push yourself to practice positive body expression and postures, the more natural it will be, plus you increase the connection between your the physical movements and your mood. In the long run, being straight and smiling even when you're not feeling like it, will ensure that you are always able to access quick energy wherever you are. The next time you're in need of an energy boost try putting your Facial Feedback Hypothesis into practice.

Its effects on brain health and mindfulness
In the last 10 years, "mindfulness" has become an increasingly popular buzzword in the psychiatry and psychology circles. It has also proven to be more than a passing trend. It has been discovered that mindfulness can result in changes to the brain which can make you to feel less stressed, keep an appropriate perspective of the situations in your life and decrease your vulnerability to depression. It also helps you make better choices and has an exciting potential for those working in many fields , such as the prevention of crime, education and social work.

What exactly is "mindfulness" refers to? In its simplest sense it's the act of paying focus on the present moment. It's about being willing to put aside worries about the future or thinking about the past. When you act mindfully it means that you are living in complete awareness of where you are today. It is possible to practice mindfulness wherever you are.

Workout: Mindful Washing Up

When you're about to wash your spoon or dish, make time to perform some mindfulness exercises. While you pour the soapy water around take note of the sensation and feel of your skin on the surface, as well as the smell of the liquid used to wash dishes as well as the noise it produces as it swirls around the bowl. Be aware of the texture of the object you're washing your hands against. If your attention is shifting, note the fact that your attention has wandered before returning it slowly but still firmly.

Mindfulness is usually associated to meditation, which is a broad term that describes the practice of focusing your attention to a specific idea, object or even your breathing. Meditation and mindfulness are not solely the domain of religious people. Though meditation is widely associated to Buddhism and Hinduism but people of all religions can gain from the practices which permit the mind to breathe.

What role does neuroplasticity play in the aspect? Studies of people who regularly meditate show that the practice of meditation can alter the brain in an approach that improves the quality of life and well-being. A report published by the journal Neuroreport stated that when compared with those who had never meditated the people who meditated regularly were more likely to have larger cortices. This was particularly evident in the parts of the brain responsible for processing sensory information and focusing concentration. (If you're looking to remember more of what you've learned and stay focused for longer in the workplace or in school it is a good option to increase your performance.)

It's not just that, the practice of long-term meditation can help you control your feelings. It doesn't mean that regular meditators are robots, but it does mean that meditation gives you the ability to keep your strong emotions under control and make more informed decision-making, controlled choices in responding to difficult situations.

Exercise: Mediation, Part I

Simple breathing is a very popular exercise for those who are new to it. All you have to do is stand or sit in a comfortable posture. Relax your eyes, and concentrate at your breathing. Keep a steady count of your breaths. Focus your attention on this seemingly simple task. If your thoughts begin to wander then bring it back to your breathing.

Exercise: Meditation, Part II

If you are unable to stay still for long periods or aren't comfortable the idea of focusing on your breathing, walking meditation might be an ideal alternative. Find a calm room or outdoor space, and then walk through the space in an unison. Make sure you keep your pace steady. Pay attention to the sensation that you feel on your feet when they come into contact with the ground.

If you begin to get into an habit of challenging negative thoughts and practicing meditation each day, you'll quickly notice that your brain is responsive to your new routines. Even though you may not be able see the changes in your brain on the MRI or PET scanner but you can be certain that your brain's ability to change will cause significant shifts in your mood and outlook. Think about how calmer and happier your life can be after you gain more control over your mood and emotional reactions! Begin by meditating for a few minutes every day, and gradually increase to 20-30 mins each in the morning or at night.

Chapter 4: Neuroplasticity And Memory

Your memory is amazing. It is almost impossible to store anything and it is sometimes able to amaze us. Have you ever had a moment of reflection and thought about an event that occurred over 10 years ago? Are you wondering what makes it so simple to recall some irrelevant information, but difficult to remember the information that is important? In this chapter, we'll guide you through everything you should know about memory.

What is the reason We Forget Things

Before we get into ways to enhance your memory, we should take a look at the causes for why you lose things at all. The main goal is while you're learning new information your brain doesn't believe that it's relevant enough to be kept in mind.

As you gain new knowledge and acquire new skills, you begin to store the experiences, skills and information into your temporary memory.

If your brain believes that it's valuable enough to remember and it's able to move these thoughts into your memory for the long run. The short-term memory of your brain will comprise of quick images that you can see tiny pieces of information that you hear, as well as other items that you get your hands on. Long-term memory will consist of a general notion of what took place in that long-term memory of your story. It will include certain details is likely to be remembered, but much of it is lost during the process. One reason why you may not be recalling details is that they're not part of your long-term memory at all.

If your brain isn't organizing things correctly, then you'll not be able to recall things accurately. To help you remember things better when you're learning there are several things. Make sure you're putting all your focus and attention on memory and keep these pieces of information in your memory. If you're learning something, ensure that you are focusing on recalling it, then you'll be able to keep it in mind for longer.

Another reason you may be having trouble recalling information is due to distraction distracting, distraction, and other factors that make it difficult to focus fully on the things you have to master.

If you are constantly distracted by other images, or people speaking about anxiety and thoughts running through your mind constantly it can be much more difficult to recall individual pieces of information. Also, we need to consider what we might be unconsciously suppressing or dissociating in the present.

Consider the last time you felt overwhelmed as you had the conversation with someone. Perhaps you thought about all the work you needed to complete and the endless list of tasks you needed to be completed that evening and all the other things that made you feel overwhelmed.

These thoughts ran through your head while someone other person was trying to communicate with you. Perhaps they were talking about schedules for your weekend. Maybe they were sharing with you an interesting story, or telling an additional information you could have kept in mind. Then, later in the week you were asked about the story, but you're not able to recall anything because you were anxious to hear to them in the first place. Sometimes, we lose connection to the present moment due to our stress.

In order to truly begin to build our memory, we must learn to be able to concentrate. It is important to master the ability to be attentive and remain focused in the present. Before we offer you suggestions for that, we need to take a look at the enormous memory that our brains have.

Your Brain's Storage

Sometimes it seems like we're in a hurry to store things in our memories. The most important thing to keep in mind is that our brain isn't the same as our wardrobe.

Your closet could be filled with boxes, but in the end, you'll be unable to fit everything in. Your brain is never running out of storagespace; you will always have more storage for your brain.

Every phone tablet, or another electronic device you've owned isn't as powerful as the amount of storage you've got in your head. You're probably able to have read every book ever been written and have room inside your brain to discover more.

The reason you can remember things is not because your brain is stuffed with memory. You may be wondering why you can recall the tune of the commercial you watched when you were only six years older, but not as well as you remember the birthday celebration of your boyfriend's mother.

However, it's not an issue of storage, nor is it that you must rid your brain. Your brain will take care of that by itself, in any case.

Your memory won't be affected by things you are aware of. Your mind will be influenced by the things you do while you're learning new knowledge. Afterward, it's essential to keep track of all the new information you've learned to ensure that you don't lose them.

Your brain seems to have unlimited storage capacity, so don't assume that this could be the reason you're not able to master certain things. Your brain's capacity to expand is endless and change and it can change its shape at any time. It's unlike a hard drive that can only do the number of things it can do.

Your memory is made of plastic and now is the perfect time to understand how to make use of the fullest extent possible.

How anxiety and depression affect Memory

The people who suffer from depression and anxiety may know how difficult it is to keep track of certain details. Let's examine a few reasons why these mental disorders may result in less active memory than others.

The primary reason why depression and anxiety could impact your memory is due to the fight or flight response. If you are in this kind of state that the fight or flight response can trigger your brain to cease trying as hard to recall things. All of your attention will focus on protecting you. Consider the last time you were in a state of extreme level of anxiety. It's likely that you don't recall it, but there's a high chance that you've experienced terrifying experiences that you only recall from another's viewpoint. This is because your brain isn't trying to process details and has put all its attention and energy on ensuring that you're vigilant to safeguard yourself as much as you can.

Another point to take into consideration is that occasionally our brain can shut down certain memories to protect us also. If you're constantly depressed, you could be constantly in a state of dissociation as it is easier for the mind to handle this rather than to deal with the terrible emotions and feelings you feel when you are depressed.

Consider the times when you find something that you don't enjoy, such as an article in the news or a disgusting video or any other similar thing You just turn away from a sense of desperation. This is exactly the way your brain works when you're anxious or depressed. It doesn't want to go through those tough emotions. If you are experiencing negative emotions, it makes you to feel depressed. It can also have adverse impacts on your body. To protect yourself from mental illness You dissociate, in order that your brain is no longer able to cope with these kinds of issues.

The most important thing to remember is that having anxiety or depression does not mean that you'll be unable to recall certain things. It's just that you have to make a more conscious effort to remember these details. In fact, stress can increase your memory when you're stressed out; it's easier to remember the little things that others might not be able to see. For instance, if you say that you're concerned about your appearance. you could pick out all the small details of your face, your clothes hairstyle, and everything else, and also other people. The best thing you can do is to keep a record of these things, and take note of those little things. Create little notes in your mind to track the little things you observe when you are in a state of anxiety.

Sometimes, these issues can set us back. However, if we're stronger than them, and can learn to manage these mental illness that will benefit us later on.

Decluttering Your Brain

As we've already mentioned the brain's capacity to never be depleted of storage and it's not as your closet, where you need to clear out old stuff in order to allow room for new. But, it could aid in decluttering your thoughts and clear them out so that your brain function at its best in the future. Let's look at some steps will help you declutter your mind to increase your neuroplasticity. One of the first things you can do is clear the physical area. You may not be aware of the importance of this because it's something that happens in the background. occurs. Your brain can be processing the information it is able to see in front of it. Imagine you're sitting at your desk before you, your computer is there as well as a cup with pen pens inside it, a pile of papers, a photo of your family as well as a lamp that you have planted and a few other things across the walls, and a couple of other items on your desk, and a few other things everywhere.

While at the same time when you're at your desk you are able to see everything out of the corner of your eyes. You're not sitting there to think about a cup, plant or mail and so elsewhere in your mind however, your brain is aware of it and picks up the details like cameras. It's using a tiny amount of your brain's power to think about these items. For the majority of us, this isn't enough to be distracting. Therefore, in an area that is shared, little decorative elements scattered around won't cause harm. But, if your space is littered with unfinished projects heaps of garbage and other things that keep you distracted from your work, this could eat the brain's energy.

For instance, let's say that you have a chair that's half painted in your room you'd like to complete. Perhaps you have a quilt that must be stitched. Maybe there's an entire dresser you have to clear. If you observe the side of the eye while working, your brain will continue to recognize this. It will always be aware of the fact that you have to take action on this, too. It'll remind you that you have something that must be accomplished.

What can you do to recall information

When you've learned how to recall things more effectively this can alter your brain. What can you do to remember the information you're learning?

Sometimes , we absorb details, and know how to save it correctly. When it's time to remember it difficult to do it. How many times you've had a conversation with someone, and perhaps they wanted to know an instance of what you're speaking about. There are a million instances in your head to reference however you are unable to recall anything for any reason. There are some options we can take to help you recall more easily. The first thing you could make is to use an anchor. A anchor will keep your attention on the event you're trying recall.

Let's say you're trying to learn names of the classmates you've met.

Five of them are Judy, Ben, Kyle, Tom, and Jessica. Every time you glance at their names, you may apply either of your hands on the table. For example, Judy, contact your thumb on the table. Speak, Ben, move your fingertip towards the table, and continue. You can say, Kyle, touch your middle finger to the table and the list goes on. If you're unable to recall the names of your friends, attempt mimicking the gesture, and you'll find that you're able to recall your names once you've learned them.

Another method to help you remember things is to use Mnemonics. This involves using the first letter of every word and linking it to something else . It could be akin to an acronym, perhaps.

Think of the program. D.A.R.E. This is a reference to education on the dangers of drug abuse. But, in the overall word, it is dare. The acronym is actually an expression that you could remember when you must remember important information such as this. It is helpful if you remember it initially, by using an acronym. Another method to remember it is to think of poems or other forms form of phrase or pattern that will aid.

Imagine the worlds. Many people used to say, "My very educated mother has just gave our nine pizzas." This was a reference to an order for the solar system: Mercury, Venus, Earth, Mars, Jupiter, Uranus, Neptune, and Pluto. Of course, we are aware the fact that Pluto has ceased to be a globe, but it was the thought that was in the back of my mind for the best way to keep in mind this important order.

Don't limit yourself to the context of education in which you are studying something academically. Be aware that it can be applied to any subject you're trying to recall from your day-to-day everyday life. It's easier to remember this information if your focus is on learning it in an innovative and simple manner in the beginning.

The Best Methods to Improve Memory

Let's take a look at couple of other practical suggestions and exercises that you could make use of to boost your memory in general.

If you're doing something, and you're taking details that must be remembered, locate another thing you could connect this to. Many people take notes using a gum or mint within their mouths. When you are ready to test yourself, you should take the same mint or chew gum and chew on it during the test. It will help you recall the facts much more easily. If you're in the process of studying, listen to classical music when you're able of listening to music while taking the exam, you can play that same music from classical. Secondary association makes it simpler to recall important information.

Another way to recall information is to build your own mental map. This puts your mind in the physical space which you can be able to associate with the information you are learning. Let's take the example of planets once more. Imagine that you're trying to recall the order. You can create mental maps in your head using an area you are familiar with. Perhaps it's the street you take a walk on every day as you head to work. It starts with your home next to your neighbors' house Then there's an church. Then you'll see a school. There's a daycare and so on.

Every location you visit will be associated with a distinct planet. When you're trying recall the planets, then later you can bring this mental map back to your mind and go through it. you'll discover that it's easier to recall important details by this method.

You could also create an actual map to aid in remembering things. You might not be so worried about recollecting information that has changed rather, you're trying to remember old facts. The first thing you should do is create an outline of the location which you're trying to recall memories of. As an example, suppose it's your mid-50s, and you don't even remember much about your childhood was like. You've had so many great memories, however, in your later years, you can't recall any of it. Start by getting an ordinary piece of paper , a pencil, or pen, relax and draw with your best memory a sketch of your home from childhood. You can draw a sketch of a sketch now. You draw your living area bedrooms, kitchen as well as an overall plan of the layout. You can then get an extra level of detail and begin sketching where furniture could be. When you've done this you'll be amazed by how much you start to recall. You can then go through every room and draw precise images and images on various pieces of paper in order to help retain even more. The brain's ability to associate things you are learning with visual models is going be the most effective method to remember information. If you are able to think of ways to visualize things yourself and increase your memory.

Chapter 5: Brain Plasticity Exercises

For you to stay healthy, it's not enough to only exercise your body. It is also essential to work your brain. For many years, some scientists believed that the brain does not develop during childhood, so we lose neurons each year until we reach the age of. But, recent research has revealed that the brain continues to make neuronal connections all throughout the course of our life, based on our experiences.

The improvement of the neuroplasticity in the brain by doing exercises for the brain will enhance the functioning and performance of your brain, despite the presence of elements that could cause damage to the brain, such as drug use, stress or alcohol, as well as aging and growth factors. Similar to doing aerobic exercises to strengthen your heart, it's crucial to keep reconditioning your brain through regular exercise for the brain.

Benefits of regular exercise for the brain

There are numerous benefits to regularly doing brain exercises, which can lead to improved cognitive function and performance. Below are the advantages of brain exercises that enhance the neuroplasticity of the brain.

The practice of brain exercises can safeguard your brain from the stress of stress. Stress has been known to decrease neural plasticity in the brain. If the brain is in a stressful state and the dimensions of the dendrites of the neurons are likely to become smaller. When neurons shrink, they reduce the synapses in the brain, decreasing connectivity between neural cells. Studies have revealed that after the stress is lessened the synapses are able to be replaced or increase in length.

Exercises in the brain can help lessen the symptoms of depression. Depression, just like stress can trigger changes in the shape of the brain which can cause them to shrink or shrink.

Exercises in the brain can also trigger the production of a variety of brain hormones that assist in improving not only mood, but also stimulate the development of neural connections, thus enhancing the neuroplasticity of the brain.

The capability for the brain of a human to heal is increased when brain-training exercises are carried out. These are the reasons why regular brain exercises is important.

Exercises for brain plasticity: Rules for the Brain

Now you're looking forward to training your brain. Before you begin it is crucial that you are aware of precautions and guidelines to ensure that you get the best out of your brain exercise. Keep in mind that neurons not properly stimulated will not connect and this will render every effort in vain. Below are the basic rules you should be aware of to ensure that you have enough stimulation to stimulate your brain.

Regularly practice. The neurons that aren't sufficiently stimulated usually do not connect. This is particularly the case when you have suffered brain injury. It is vital to start practicing neuroplasticity exercises before your neurons begin to cease to function. If you regularly practice you will not only see the neural connections strengthen, but also your neurons will be rejuvenated according to numerous studies.

The exercises must be well-balanced. It is essential to note that repeated brain exercises over a long period of instances can result in stimulation of brain cells that are located in the targeted regions. When this happens, it can leads to the squeeze out of the data from the new neural connections that are being made in other brain regions that may not be required for brain function.

Seek out improvement in your everyday functioning. You can improve your brain connections through brain-based games but if your only gain exercise from these games, you'll not be able to continuously keep your brain active. It is essential to incorporate brain-training exercises into your everyday activities so that , even when you're performing simple routines or tasks your brain is continuously being stimulated.

Beware of certain exercises available on the marketplace. There are a lot of brain games that are advertised in the name of neuroplasticity training. Although they are marketed as such, it's important to be aware that the majority of these activities aren't really efficient. Be sure to practice neuroplasticity exercises that have been proven to work.

How can you improve brain Plasticity

The process of improving the neuroplasticity in your brain does not require expensive and complicated brain games. There are a variety of different types of brain exercises that can be done to are suitable for your lifestyle without having to shell out money. This article will go over the various types of brain exercises that you can perform to strengthen the neural connections you have throughout your day-to-day life.

Intellectual activities: Engaging in activities that provide stimulation to the brain could provide the physical exercise you need to strengthen your brain. There are numerous intellectual activities you can take part in to increase the speed of your neural connections . These include playing board games, participating in debates , or taking online classes.

Make your tasks more interesting It's true that normal activities can challenge your brain by performing tasks that are different from your normal job. For example, if you typically hike on a standard trail, it is possible to discover a new route to explore. What happens to the brain once you introduce variety to your work is that you expand the capabilities of your brain through creating a variety of activities.

Engage in physical activities: Engaging in physical exercises can bring a host of advantages for your brain health. One of the main reasons for taking part in physical exercise is essential for neuroplasticity is that it helps the brain release brain-stimulating hormones. The research has revealed that stroke patients who engage in exercises for rehabilitation can stimulate neurons. When they do gentle exercises, such as walking, it may strengthen the neural connections connected to move.

Participate in brainwave entertainment Brainwave entertainments are based on the use of invisible waves to stimulate the brain. It has been discovered that binaural beats may stimulate brain activity in both the right and left brain hemispheres, which can boost brain thought. Binaural beats are defined as frequencies below 1000 and 1500 in frequency. They affect the functioning of the brain via the process known as "frequency subsequent response" which stimulates various locations in the brain. What are the best places to hear binaural beats? There are a variety of ways to engage in brainwave entertainment . For instance, the listening of meditation songs, sounds of nature , and the rustling of the leaves from wind are among the brainwave sources can be used to enhance your brain's connection.

Meditate: Meditation can improve brain health by reducing anxiety. Because meditation also increases levels of the hormones within the brain, it may aid in improving ability to make decisions, memory and the ability to focus. Through research conducted by researchers they've discovered that people who regularly engage in meditation have higher cognitive functions due to the growth of the gyri. These are the folds that appear on the top of the brain.

Consume omega-3 rich fatty acid food items: Consuming brain-friendly foods like those with plenty in Omega-3 fats could lower the chance of suffering from hemorrhagic stroke. Research has also revealed that omega-3 fatty acid-rich foods may increase the concentration of a variety of molecules, including that of the neurotrophic factor in brains (BNDF) to increase neurons' neuroplasticity. This molecule is able to regulate the development, survival and differentiation of nerve cells.

Consume other foods that boost your brain Apart from eating food that are rich in omega-3 fatty acids It is also essential to consume green leafy vegetables since they are rich in minerals and vitamins that help aid in the prevention of the onset of dementia. It is also important to incorporate nuts to your diet as they're loaded with zinc which has been proven to boost cognitive abilities. Zinc has been proven to regulate the plasticity of synapses as well as safeguard the brain from free radicals. Other food items that you have to consume include foods that are high in folate acid Vitamin B12, vitamin folic acid and complex carbohydrates since they boost the cognitive capacity of the brain, keeping out the possibility of developing cerebral infarcts.

Coffee consumption has lots of benefits to those who wish to enhance their brain's ability to adapt. They are a source of natural stimulants that stimulate the sympathetic nervous system that is the component of the brain responsible for speeding up the cognitive functions. Also, they contain antioxidants that help to restore neurons following injury or stress. Studies have shown that drinking eight ounces of black tea can enhance short-term memory as well as concentration span.

Do some backpacking when you travel, make sure to carry a backpack so you'll be capable of observing how the city streets are laid out in your city you're visiting. Studies of neuroimaging show that those who backpack exhibit better spatial memory, compared to those who depend on the tour guide. It is because backpacking can help you exercise your brain, and in the process you can enjoy your trip.

Chewing gum boosts mental function, mood and long-term focus, as per the Center for Occupational and Health Psychology at Cardiff University. What's more, whenever you chew on gum it enhances your mental alertness as well as reduces stress.

Exercise to build muscles The use of weights for exercise is not just helpful in getting your muscles stronger but will also enhance your cognitive capabilities. According to a study by scientists from the Psychobiology and Exercise Research

Center in Brazil muscle building can boost the brain-derived neurotrophic factor which regulates the development and survival in brain cells. If you do lift weights, ensure that you're not only exercising your muscles, but also boost the function of your brain.

Doodling is an unproductive activity, but numerous experts believe that doing doodling is an effective method to stimulate your brain. Doodling is not just a way to keep your brain active but aids in strengthening neural connections.

Allow your mind to wander Many people are afraid of their minds from wandering. It's not a bad thing and many experts suggest that letting your mind wander for just short amounts of time can boost your imagination and solving problems. Researchers from the Department of Psychological and Brain Sciences at the University of California found out that mind wandering that is prospective can enhance memory and also stimulate the autobiographical plan. If you are wandering about, then allow it to be. It's a normal behavior and good for your brain too.

Reduce your intake of calories: Numerous studies have shown that reducing your calories intake doesn't just help you lose weight, but can also decrease the chance of developing of neurodegenerative diseases. Researchers from Massachusetts Institute of Technology noted that rats that have been in laboratory experiments have a 30% higher chance of improving their learning and memory skills. If you are a person with a low calorific intake, it triggers the enzyme known as Sirtuin 1. It protects the brain from diseases caused by age.

Have fun often: Laughing often does not only relieve anxiety and depression, but it could also boost the level of Oxygen that the brain produces. Research has shown that people who are happy throughout their lives have higher cognitive abilities than those who suffer from melancholy.

Play video games The video games are addicting, however there are advantages from playing videogames. Studies have shown that people that play games experience higher levels of visual selective awareness and more accurate reaction times and speed in completing real-life tasks. Therefore, playing video games isn't just an activity that is only enjoyed by the elite, but an excellent way to increase the brain's ability to adapt.

Chess is a game that is known for a long time as a well-known mind game. Many studies have demonstrated the benefits of chess playing among children. Chess-playing children showed increased math and language abilities.

More books to read Read more books: Reading helps keep your brain functioning. But, it doesn't necessarily mean only reading things that you love. If you wish to maintain your brain's health by reading, you should be sure to read challenging books that stimulate the brain. Many neuroscientists advise reading mysteries because they are filled with intricate plots due to the mystery in the story.

Add spice to your meals Consuming foods that are spicy could assist in maintaining memory and also increase cognitive functioning. It is because spice contains polyphenols which possess antioxidant properties in nature that help protect our nervous system. Some examples of spices you should consider include cumin, cinnamon and sage. Also, cilantro and sage are fantastic for memory enhancement, so ensure that you dust your food items with these components.

Use any musical instrument you want whether it's an instrument like a guitar or a keyboard playing instruments that are musical is not just fun, it's also an excellent method to improve the neural connections you have. Research done on brains belonging to musicians showed that the gray matter in musicians exhibit profound multiregional differences when compared with those who don't play music. This is a sign of their higher capacity to long-term memory and learning.

Yoga can not just improve your physical health, however it also improves your mental and spiritual wellbeing. A number of studies have demonstrated that yoga practices can boost the levels of GABA in the brain. GABA is a hormone that fights depression as well as other mood disorders.

Get plenty of water in your system your brain will not perform as it should if you're dehydrated. Apart from providing brain oxygen, it aids in maintaining the balance of fluids in the brain. Without proper fluid balance the brain can't transmit impulses create neurotransmitters or release hormones.

A good night's sleep Insuffering yourself with enough sleep will allow you to perform better in your cognitive and behavioral functions. Furthermore, it's important in enhancing your cognitive abilities as well as mood, concentration and focus. However researchers are also highlighting how important it is to have naps in order to increase your focus and memory.

Find solutions to puzzles. The brain needs stimulation all the time. Playing simple games of puzzles such as Sudoku and crosswords may boost the flow of oxygen and glucose consumption in the brain. Additionally, it helps release dopamine, which in turn stimulates the development of brain cells.

Self-hypnosis: Altering your thinking process and understanding how to shift your focus using self-hypnosis is a great way to gain a more focused and sharper in their thinking. It can also to increase your tolerance for discomfort and also increase your concentration when trying new things.

Learning a language Learn a new language: Learning a new language can do wonders to your brain. Research has shown that people who speak two languages are less likely to develop dementia when compared to those who speak only one language. The reason is, when we are introduced to an additional language or a foreign language, the brain will get so stimulated that they fire up signals that increase the speed of neural connections.

Maintain a positive and healthy relationship. How can nurturing a positive relationships aid individuals in having greater neuroplasticity? Social inadequacies resulting from unbalanced relationships can trigger anxiety and stress which can lead in a variety of cognitive problems, including decline in cognition. Studies have shown that older people with a strong social networks have lower rates of cognitive decline when compared with those who have weak relationships with others.

Engage in a conversation that is enjoyable Engaging in a good conversation can boost your memory and cognitive performance. Psychologists from Michigan's University of Michigan noted that conversations with others create positive relationships, which could result in improved cognitive performance and improved mood.

Get your stuff organized Sorting out your stuff not just good for your body, but it is also good for your brain. If you organize your belongings and organizing your belongings, you'll be able to increase your cognitive abilities as it refocuses your mind about the places you place your belongings which improves your memory.

Handwriting is a method of writing: Many people do not realize the many advantages of writing handwritten letters. Handwriting helps individuals build kinesthetic perception which will enable the brain to efficiently process information. Researchers have discovered that finger movements in response to handwriting trigger the larger brain regions. This brain region is associated with language, memory and thinking.

Say it loudly The act of speaking things out loud can be beneficial to the brain. Speaking aloud helps enhance our memory. If you're preparing to take an examination, make sure you do not just mumble words, but do it loudly.

Positive thinking: Thinking positive can help your brain become more positive, thereby increasing the brain's capacity to acquire and learn new skills.

Quitting smoking cigarettes removes your brain of Oxygen as well as fills the brain up with carbon monoxide and free radicals. This reduces your cognitive capacity due to injuries to the lining of blood vessels in the brain. It also increases the risk of developing strokes and cancer.

Avoid alcohol and alcohol: People who drink alcohol and use drugs can affect their perception, judgment, and control. The consumption of alcohol and drugs may also deprive the brain of Oxygen and produce a large amount of free radicals in the body, thereby preventing the development and development of synapses.

There are a variety of things you can try to boost your brain's plasticity. It isn't just engaging in brain exercises that improve your brain's performance. Maintaining a healthy and balanced lifestyle with exercises for the brain can help improve neural connections as well as stimulate brain synapses.

Chapter 6: Incredible Human Brain's Capacity Brain

The conventional wisdom has was that we were already born with neurons, which we could require throughout the course all of life. (Neurons are brain cells that process and transmits information to one the other through electrical signals or chemical signals that essentially creates responses in the body.)

We were also led believed that the circuits in the brain that connects these neurons , which allows the body's system to act and react to any internal or external stimuli has been fixed in place in the beginning of our lives. It is believed that it is difficult to learn new things and develop new skills in the last few years of life. The conventional wisdom led us to think that our brain gets rigid and static in the adulthood, without newly formed brain cells (neurons) being created and old cells dying as we get older.

However, this knowledge is now considered to be outdated because of the evidence that has been uncovered that proves the fact that neurogenesis (the neural process in the brain that creates neurons by progenitors cells as well as neural stem cells) in human beings occurs not just in the childhood years but also throughout life (i.e. from the moment of birth until death). This could mean only that no one will ever become too old be able to learn new tricks or learn new techniques because new neurons will be around to facilitate the process.

What is increasingly fascinating and useful, especially for teachers and parents are the numerous research studies that show that the neurons that are already in existence and ones that are created can undergo changes in their structure as well as function depending on how people actively interact with their environment. It is only one possible meaning is that we could reinvent our brains by the choices we make about what we will do to the objects we encounter.

A significant discovery that recent studies on neural function have revealed is that the brain can regenerate itself but also organize and repair itself in order to handle injuries or diseases to the brain. The brain of the human being tries to ensure that our organs are functioning at their the highest level. When certain brain cells fail because of injuries or diseases It identifies ways to keep them functioning normally by shifting the tasks to be completed by affected brain cells unaffected brain cells.

The brain's remarkable capacity to continually regenerate itself the capacity of learning or unlearn and then revisit things based on an person's preference response, as well as the capacity to reorganize and reconfigure the neural networks it has as a result of experiences and learning are all part of the umbrella of brain science referred to as neuroplasticity. Due to the vast implications of this rapidly developing field of science for our lives neuroplasticity is now one of the areas of most intriguing research studies of the present.

What exactly is Neuroplasticity?

Neuroplasticity can be used to describe the inherent characteristic of the brain to change the structure of its neurons and alter the connections in its neural networks as a result of different factors such as brain development, the new information that is thrown at it or stimulation of the sensory organs, and damage or diseases that affect certain neurons. It's also known by terms like neural plasticity or brain plasticity.

The term"neuroplasty" was first used in the year 1948 in the work of Professor Dr. Jerry Konorski, a neurophysiologist from Polish Descent. (Perhaps the reason for choosing the term "plasticity" is an expression of the unique quality of malleable plastic – it is able to be made to any shape or size you like once heated.) In the past, the notion that brains are plastic was only a thought that the majority of medical field pondered with their mouths pressed against their lips. It was merely a idea without the benefit of thorough research and work to prove it.

The brain's ability to change is not a new idea however. In 1793, Michele Vicenzo Malacarne, an Italian anatomist, in an experiment that he conducted with laboratory animals, realized that the brain wasn't an unchanging, rigid structure like many believed. He examined the brains of a pair of animals that were extensively trained prior to his study and compared them to brains of two untrained animals. He observed that the cerebellums of two animals that were trained are considerably larger than the animals that were not trained, indicating that the brain develops with the training. But, no one was aware of its significance findings at the time and his findings were shortly discarded to the dustbin of the past.

Nearly a century after that in 1890, to be precise, researcher named Dr. William James once again presented the same notion that the brain and its functions can be fixed in our adulthood in the book Principles of Psychology which was published that same year. However, once again the medical establishment just shrugged it off.

It was another 33 years until another study proving the brain's plasticity out. In 1923, Karl Lashley experimented with monkeys to demonstrate that the brain can be able to form new neural pathways following the existing ones were shut down or damaged. Yet, as always, the most of the brain scientists at the period weren't enthused by the idea , and were unaware of the vast implications of his study.

It wasn't until the late 1960's that the neuroscientist community across the globe began to pay attention to the notion that brains are plastic. The myriad of evidences collected from a variety of research and experiments done by other world-renowned brain researchers (like Michael Merzenich) was able to fill the newswires as well as medical journal with undeniable evidence that neuroplasticity exists.

In the present, Neuroplasticity has ceased to be a mere notion. It's now a definite fact of life , the knowledge of which can open up a wide range of possibilities to enhance the quality of our lives. It's not surprising that brain researchers and scientists today burn out the oil lamps , searching for new methods to utilize this newly discovered information. All of them have been bitten by the neuroplasticity virus. It's not surprising that educators and parents are savoring every neuroplasticity-related materials they can get their fingertips on. First of all they owe it the children to equip them with the best brains that they can to ensure their future. Researchers who are working on a brain-computer interface that could be utilized by those who have impaired senses have discovered immense value in the advancements made in the field of neuroplasticity, using their knowledge of this emerging science as the basis to their work. The growing understanding of neuroplasticity helps medical professionals. Their understanding and perception shift regarding neuroplasticity provided them with the chance to investigate different ways to treat brain injury caused by strokes and to handle other medical conditions like emotional disorders, chronic pain as well as psychopathic conditions. There is no doubt that any research on the brain using neuropathy will provide improved treatments and management of clinical instances involving the brain.

Chapter 7: Brain-Boosting Exercise Tips

Although mental exercise is essential to maintain brain health, it does not mean that you don't need to work out. Physical activity aids in keeping your brain alert. It improves the oxygen supply to your brain, and lowers the chance of developing disorders which can lead to loss of memory including heart disease and diabetes. Exercise also increases the effect of beneficial brain chemicals and lowers stress hormones. In addition, exercise is an essential factor in neuroplasticity, by stimulating development factors, and engaging the development of new neural connections.

Exercise tips for brain health

Aerobic exercise is particularly beneficial for brain health So, make sure you choose activities that help to keep your blood flowing. All that helps your heart is good to your brain.

Do you take a long time to let go of the fog of sleep when you get up? If so, you could be surprised to discover that doing some exercise early in the morning before you get started on your day makes a an enormous difference. Along with clearing the dust, it helps you to be prepared for the day.

Activities with hand eye coordination or advanced motor skills are beneficial to brain development.

The benefits of exercise breaks are that they aid in overcoming depression and slumps in the afternoon. Even a quick stroll or a few Jacks could be enough to refresh your brain.

If you're experiencing traumatizing anxiety or you are trapped in unhealthy, repetitive behavior...

...Try working out the muscles that are connected to fighting or flight with focus. Exercises that require both legs and arms and that are done in a way that is focused and with an awareness of your emotional and physical experience are particularly effective at decreasing the effects of trauma. Activities like running, walking and swimming, or rock-climbing are a great way to stimulate your senses and increase your awareness of others and yourself, when you do them with a focus.

There's a huge distinction between the amount of sleep you can go in comparison to the quantity you require to be at your best. It is a fact that more than 95% of people need at least 7.5 or 9 hours rest each at night to avoid sleeping insufficiency. Even slacking off the amount of time you sleep can make some difference! The ability to think creatively, memory, problem-solving skills and critical thinking abilities are all weakened.

Sleep is essential for learning and memory in an the most fundamental of ways. Studies have shown that sleep is essential to consolidate memory as well as the primary memory-enhancing activities occurring in the deepest levels of sleep.

Make sure you are on a regular sleeping routine. Sleep every night at the exact time each evening and rise every morning.

Do not alter your routine, not even on holidays and weekends.

Be sure to stay away from screens for at the very least an hour prior to bedtime. The blue light that is emitted by devices like TVs, tablets phones, computers and TVs cause you to wake up and reduce hormones, such as melatonin. These can make you sleepy.

Cut back on caffeine. Caffeine has different effects on people. Some people are very sensitive to caffeine, and morning coffee can affect sleeping in the evening. Reduce your consumption or removing it entirely If you suspect that it's keeping you awake.

Tip 4: Create time for your friends

When you consider ways to improve your memory are you thinking of "serious" tasks like taking on puzzles like the New York Times crossword puzzle or learning chess strategies, or are there more casual activities like hanging out with your friends or watching a humorous film that comes to thoughts? If you're like the majority of us, then it's the latter. Numerous studies have shown that having a full life of people you love and having fun can bring cognitive advantages.

Healthy relationships can be the most effective brain booster

Humans are extremely social creatures. We're not designed to live or even thrive in solitude. Interactions with others stimulate our brains. fact, being in contact with other people could be the most effective form of brain workout.

Research has shown that having meaningful friendships as well as an effective support system are crucial not only for mental health, but also for the health of your brain. In a recent study conducted by the Harvard School of Public Health For instance the researchers found that people who were the most relationships had the lowest rate of decline in memory.

There are many options to take advantage of the brain's benefits and the memory-enhancing advantages of socializing. Join a club, volunteer or make it a priority to meet with friends more frequently or even call on the phone. If you're not helpful, don't ignore the importance of having pets, particularly the extremely social dog.

Tip 5: Manage the stress level under control

Stress is among the brain's most feared enemies. As time passes, chronic stress damages brain cells and causes damage to the hippocampus. This is the brain's region that is involved in the creation of new memories as well as retrieval of older ones. Research has been linked to stress and memory loss.

Tips to manage stress

Be realistic about your expectations (and be ready to refuse!)

Make breaks throughout the day

Let your emotions out instead of making them into a bottle

Create a balanced balance between your work and leisure time

Concentrate on one thing at one time, and not trying to do multiple tasks at once.

The memory-enhancing, stress-busting benefits of meditation

The evidence-based research supporting the benefits to mental health of meditation keeps piling up. Research shows that meditation can to treat a variety of illnesses, such as anxiety, depression chronic pain, diabetes and hypertension. Meditation can also increase focus, concentration and creativity, memory as well as reasoning and learning abilities.

Meditation creates its "magic" by altering the structure of the brain. Brain scans reveal regular meditators have higher stimulation in the prefrontal area of their brains an part of the brain that is associated with happiness and tranquility. Meditation also improves the thickness of cerebral cortex as well as increases the connectivity between neurons, all of which enhances mental clarity and memory abilities.

Sixth Tip: Make a good laugh

It's been said that laughing is the best medicine which is also for the brain as well as the memory and also for the body. Contrary to emotional responses that are restricted to specific regions within the brain laughing activates many regions of the brain.

Additionally, watching jokes and thinking up punch lines can stimulate areas of the brain that are essential for creativity and learning. According to psychotherapist Daniel Goleman notes in his book Emotional Intelligence "laughter appears to aid people think more widely and communicate more easily."

Are you looking for ways to create more joy to your daily life? Start by learning these fundamentals:

You can laugh at yourself. Talk about your embarrassing moments. One of the best ways to treat yourself more seriously would be to share those times we took ourselves too seriously.

If it is obvious that you are laughing, you should move towards it. The majority of the time, people are extremely pleased to share a funny story because they get to laugh to feed the laughter that you can find. If you hear laughter take a look and attempt to participate.

Enjoy time with fun, lively people. They are the kind of people who can be found laughing easily, both at themselves as well as at life's absurdities. They are also able to discover humor in ordinary situations. Their jovial perspective and laughter is infectious.

Set yourself up with reminders to keep you motivated. Have a toy at the desk, or inside your vehicle. Make a funny posters in the office. Pick a computer screen saver that will make you smile. Capture photos of you and your family members having enjoyable.

Be attentive to children and try to emulate them. They are the best at playing, having fun and having fun.

Tip 7: Eat a brain-boosting diet

As your body requires energy, so does the brain. You've probably heard that a diet consisting of vegetables, fruits as well as whole grains "healthy" fats (such as olive oil or nuts, seafood) and lean proteins will offer a variety of health benefits. However, such diets also can enhance memory. To ensure brain health it's not only about what you eat , it's also what you do not eat. These tips on nutrition can help you boost your brain power and decrease your chances of developing dementia:

Get your omega-3s. Research has shown that omega-3 fat acids are especially beneficial to brain health. Fish is a very abundant source of omega-3, and particularly cold-water "fatty fish" like salmon and tuna, halibut, mackerel, trout, sardines and herring.

In the event that you're not a big fan of seafood, look at other sources of omega-3s like walnuts, seaweed ground flaxseed and flaxseed oil winter squash, kidneys as well as pinto beans. Also, consider spinach pumpkin seeds, broccoli and soybeans.

Reduce the amount of calories and saturated fats. Research has shown that diets that are high of saturated fat (from sources like whole milk, red meat cheese, butter cream, cheese, and Ice cream) increase the chance of developing dementia and can affect your mental focus and memory.

Consume more fruits and vegetables. Produce is loaded with antioxidants. They are substances which protect brain cells from harm. The vibrant fruits and vegetables are excellent antioxidant "superfood" sources.

Drink green tea. Green tea is a rich source of polyphenols, powerful antioxidants that shield against free radicals which can harm brain cells. Alongside other benefits drinking regularly green tea can improve mental and memory alertness as well as reduce the rate of brain aging.

Consume wines (or the juice of a grape) in moderate amounts. Making sure you keep your alcohol consumption within a reasonable range is crucial because alcohol can kill brain cells. However, when used when consumed in moderate amounts (around 1 glass per day for women and two glasses for men) drinking alcohol can enhance memory and cognitive. The red wine seems to be the most beneficial option, because it's high in resveratrol, which is a flavonoid which increases the flow of blood within the brain, and decreases the chance of developing Alzheimer's disease. Other sources of resveratrol include cranberry juice, grape juice fresh berries and grapes as well as peanuts.

Tip 8: Recognize and treat health issues

Are you feeling that your memory has experienced an unexpected decline? If so, there could be a medical or lifestyle issue that is that is to be the cause.

It's not only dementia or Alzheimer's disease that cause memory loss. There are many illnesses that affect mental health, and medications that affect memory:

Heart disease and risk factors. Cardiovascular disease and risk factors for it like high cholesterol and blood pressure are associated with mild cognitive impairment.

Diabetes. Studies have shown that people suffering from diabetes suffer from a greater cognitive decline than people who aren't affected by the condition.

Hormone imbalance. Menopausal women typically experience memory problems when estrogen levels decrease. For men, testosterone levels that are low may cause problems. Thyroid imbalances can cause confusion, forgetfulness, or even confusion.

Medications. A variety of prescription and over-the-counter medicines can hinder the development of clarity and memory. Common causes include allergies and cold medications as well as sleep aids and antidepressants. Discuss with your doctor or pharmacist about the possibility of adverse consequences.

Is it depression?

Troubles with emotions can take as severe a toll your brain's health as do physical issues. Indeed, mental problems with concentration, sluggishness and forgetfulness are all common signs of depression. Memory issues can be especially severe for older individuals with depression to the point that they are often misinterpreted as dementia. The positive side is that once depression is treated, memory will get back to normal.

Tip 9: Take concrete steps to help support learning and memory

Pay pay attention. You won't be able to recall something if you haven't learned about it. Likewise, you won't discover something new that will in your brain if it doesn't pay enough concentration to it. It takes around eight seconds of focused attention to encode a bit of information into your brain. When you're frequently distracted select a quiet area that isn't a distraction.

Engage as many of your senses as you can. Try to connect information to textures, colors scents, tastes, and colors. Rewriting information helps to imprint it into your brain. Even If you're a visual learner Read aloud what you'd like to keep in mind. If you can repeat it with a rhythm, that's even better.

Connect information with what you already are aware of. Link new information to data that you've already recalled regardless of whether it's a new piece of information that is based on your the previous knowledge or as basic as the address of a person who lives in a neighborhood that you know.

For more complicated information, concentrate on understanding the fundamental concepts instead of memorizing specific particulars. Try explaining your ideas to others using your own words.

Review the material you've already learned. Re-examine what you've learned on the day you first learn it, and then at intervals throughout the course of. This "spaced practice" is far more effective than cramming and is especially effective for keeping the lessons you've learned.

Utilize mnemonic devices in order to help you remember information more easily. The mnemonics (the beginning "m" can be silent) are clues of every type that aid us in remembering things, typically because they help us connect the information we need to remember by using a visual illustration, a sentence or a phrase.

Six types of mnemonic devices

Visual image. You can associate a visual with a name or a word to make it easier to remember them. Images that are pleasant, positive, are vibrant, vibrant and three-dimensional are more easy to remember. Example: To recall names like Rosa Parks and what she's most well-known for, imagine an image of a woman on a bench in a park, in a garden of roses, waiting for her bus to pull up.

Acrostic (or sentence) Create sentences in which the initial letter of each word is either part of or is the first of what you would like to keep in mind. Example of a sentence is "Every good boy is a star" to remember those lines in the treble Clef, that represents the notes G B, G D, and F.

Acronyms An acronym is a word made by taking the initial letters of the most important concepts or words you have to recall and making new words from the letters. Example: "HOMES" is a word that means "HOMES" to refer to all the words that are part of the Great Lakes: Huron, Ontario, Michigan, Erie and Superior.

Rhymes and alliteration Rhymes or alliteration (a repetition of a sounds or even syllables) or jokes can be remembered to recall more everyday details and numbers. Example A rhyme is

"Thirty days have September March, April, June along with November" to recall the seasons of the year, with just 30 days.

Method of loci: Imagine placing the things you wish to keep in mind along a path that you're familiar with or in particular locations in a room you are familiar with or structure. For example, for your shopping list, picture bananas in the foyer of your house, a pool of milk on the floor of the couch eggs descending the staircase, and bread lying on your mattress.

As you are aware. the brain is not made of plastic...Neuroplasticity, or brain plasticity, refers to the brain's ability to CHANGE throughout life.

The human brain is awe-inspiring in its ability to change its structure by forming new connections among neurons (neurons).

Along with genetic aspects as well as the environment in which the person lives, and the choices made by each individual are a major factor in the development of plasticity.

Neuroplasticity is a process that occurs in the brain...

1. At the start in life, the embryonic brain begins to organize itself.

2. In the event injuries to the brain: make up for diminished functions or increase the remaining functions.

3- Throughout adulthood: when something new is learned , it is stored in memory

Learning, plasticity and memory

Chapter 8: Exercises for the Brain that are Recommended

Don't be afraid to stretch and train your brain to its limits. Do not be reluctant to do exercises because you believe that your brain can't handle these exercises. It is really beneficial to test your reflexes and memory, as well as increase your ability to think on your feet.

Try different brain-training activities and games that will aid your brain in processing information faster and more effectively. These brain-training exercises as well as games will allow you to focus better and complete multiple tasks easily and improve the speed of your brain's reflection. They certainly help the overall mental health of your brain.

Some of the most commonly used activities for the brain are the tests for brain reflection memory test, brain reflection test, and a test of brain creativity. The test of brain reflection is simple but efficient. It is designed to test your brain's reflection by determining how quick your reflexes are.

Memory test can help you enhance memories by stimulating different areas of your brain which are responsible to retrieve and store information. This test will test your capacity to retain images.

The test for brain creativity stimulates the brain's areas to stimulate your brain's ability to think creatively. Similar exercises include brain stretching as well as Sudoku stimulants for the brain. The brain stretching game involves Sudoku, also known as the Tower of Hanoi, a game that aims to transfer discs between poles to the next.

Sudoku brain stimulation is based on Sudoku, a popular game that requires you to arrange the numbers in a particular order. This game of strategy is great to train and stimulate your brain.

It is also possible to improve the health of your brain by enhancing math and spatial thinking and brain-focused education, IQ booster, and Arrange game. Arrange is a game that is very like Sudoku since you are forced to arrange the numbers in a certain order, however in the shortest time that is possible.

Spatial intelligence is the process of using of a Rubik's-cube puzzle. It's extremely challenging as a result it stimulates many parts that are in your brain get stimulated including spatial intelligence as well as visual memory.

Problems with math require you solve many math problems as complex as you can within just a few minutes. The brain-focused game is exactly the same. The higher the difficulty level you select the more stimulated your brain gets. This game will test your brain's ability to focus.

Through the training in cognitive, you'll be able to improve your cognitive and prediction skills as well as improve your observation capabilities. This is because it involves a ball is difficult to detect quickly. The IQ booster is a chess game which can boost your abilities by allowing you to develop imaginative strategies.

Additionally is that you can also practice cross crawling or brain buttons. Cross crawling is a type of brain exercise that will help you improve your listening, spelling writing, reading and comprehension abilities by coordinating both parts of the brain. Brain buttons however can boost circulation of blood to the brain, which enhances your learning, attention and performance.

Chapter 9: Popular Myths About Human Memory

A myriad of myths have been floating around the human mind since the beginning of time in the diasporas of psychology. We all fall prey to these illogical beliefs and adhere to the prevailing beliefs without knowing the truth or even trying to discover the truth. There are many myths, one of which is religious, traditional, and are extremely difficult to overcome or change.

Some of us is of the opinion that memory power cannot be improved. However, the reality is that memory strength can be improved if you keep up a consistent, systematic routine. Continuous practice is sure to be beneficial, and people can boost the quality of their memory recall ability.

Let's discuss some of the more well-known stories about human memory.

Myth No. 1: Memory from photographs

Let's reduce the truth. There isn't a photography memory and it's highly unlikely that there is an image-based memory. In reality, that it is a method through which people improve their memory at a high level, allowing them that allows them to remember the memories with photographic accuracy. There are some people who claim to possess a photographic memory did not have the training in science to master memory retrieval. However, they might have come up with a basic version of a memory retrieval system that is similar or even similar to the best practice for memory retrieval. When we examine them in depth we will see that they have an order to keep and retrieve data.

Myth No. 2: Memory training and obsliteration

It is a fact that nobody forgets any information. In reality, all information remains in memory, even if we're unable to retrieve it. The people who train to learn to recall information will be unable to recall information. However, those who have been trained can remember more quickly than people with no formal training. The power of memory isn't fixed, if you are not using your memory abilities, naturally, you'll lose your ability to remember. A systematic practice is necessary to maintain the progress of improving your memory skills.

Myth No. 3 The concept of memory is that it is a matter

Memory isn't an issue or physical organ that you are able to recognize. It is actually a bodily organ, and it is easily identified. In reality, memory is the process, or a sequence of the process that aids in storing and then reproduce the information in textual, visual audio, sense, and emotional format, in a group or individually. Memory is a possible stage of the brain with numerous storage and sub-storage segments, and there isn't a specific location within the memory that can be identified as which memory is using to keep. Different types of data are stored in different areas in the brain.

Myth No. 4: Shortcut to remember

There is no quick way to master. Memory is a skill that can be developed by everyone, provided that they are able practice it regularly and regularly. Thus, those with natural memory might have acquired the ability to retrieve memories without any understanding about memory retention. It is possible to think that he is an individual with a remarkable capacity for memory. However, the reality is that he may have developed a method to organize and chunk information into his mind that does the trick. If you practice memory strategies in a systematic manner and with a scientific basis the process will be much easier for you.

Myth No. 5: Overuse will diminish the memory

It is not possible to disprove the idea that using memory too much could reduce the effectiveness of memory. Actually, a systematic approach to training will improve to improve the quality of memory recall ability.

Myth No. 6: Excessive memory training can boost memory power

It's another legend. Training in systematic manner can boost power of memory. There is a distinction in class between training that is excessive as well as systematic learning. The excess training will not increase or decrease the capacity of memory. Instead of attempting to train memory in an uninformed manner make sure you train scientifically and consistently. It will certainly increase your memory capacity.

Myth No. 7: We're only using 10% of memory

There isn't a way to assess this claim. There is no doubt that a large portion of us won't be utilising the entire amount of the memory. Training can help us enhance the quality of our memory. As it is possible to achieve the goal of training in memory the amount of value regardless of whether it exists or not is not important.

Myth No. 8: A lot of load can weaken your memory.

The capacity to store data in memory is not in any relationship to the quantity of information stored inside your memory. If you're not able to find the information you need, it is likely that you are not storing the information in a well-organized and systematic way. The brain is able to store the inexhaustible amount of information. The most important thing is the method it stores the memory. There isn't any space in the brain where you could fill it. This is because you're putting the data into your memory fragments.

Myth No. 9 A few people suffer from poor memory

There is no such thing as a good and bad memory. Its quality is contingent on the process you use to store the information within the brain. If you keep the data in a well-organized manner it will be easy to find.

Myth No. 10: The memories of petrifying can be repressed and retrieved in the years to come

It's a mythical notion. People are unable to forget their petrifying memories. But, the intensity of the emotion may decrease over time. In addition, they might not be able to remember the event, however the victim won't remember the particular sequence of events.

Chapter 10: Brain Training: Top 20 Powerful Techniques

Once you've got an in-depth understanding of neuroplasticity and how the brain develops over time and over time, let's cut right straight to the point and take an overview of the methods that can help improve memory and critical thinking.

Our first choice is Tetris. The original computer game may be more straightforward than the majority of puzzle games nowadays However, tests conducted by a clinical psychologist have revealed that players who played Tetris regularly had an increase in the gray matter of the brain as well as improved thinking, compared to people who did not play the game. The study found it was possible to play the game for 30 minutes a day for three months affected the brain structure of the participants. The brains of the participants revealed structural changes in the areas that are associated with movement, critical thinking reasoning, language, and processing.

Mind maps can help to increase your memory. Mind maps can be a powerful tool that allows you to investigate and consider the idea, problem or even a job. If you're in the process of learning or studying something new, take a moment to contemplate for a few minutes and then create a your mind map. It's a fantastic learning method that makes use of your brain's maximum capacity. Because mind maps aren't linear, which means you cannot study it in a linear manner It becomes a plan with all the essential details. The brain thus saves information stored in your long-term memory rather than your short-term memory which is highly unstable.

The Journey Method is a method used to help your brain become more adept at recalling lists of things. In this exercise, you will need to recall the items on your list in a way that is based on the journey you visualize in your head. It is a mnemonic link system that allows your brain to create new neural pathways after affixing them with the previous ones. If you're trying to recall an item think of a trip through all the places you've already been to (the ones that are important to you, or where you can remember them with a lot of fondness) and then associate every item on the list to the place that you would like to visit. Because your brain can quickly absorb visual information, it becomes easier for you to keep a list of things when they are linked with pictures and memories of places you've been to. This technique is only effective when you imagine the journey prior to the trip and can pinpoint a location or reference point in your mind.

Pegging is an additional method which can help improve the memory of your brain. If you're finding recalling the process of journeying difficult, this workout could also improve the memory regions of your brain. Pegging is about combining previously known facts with new information you wish to recall. In this case, you're mentally putting your data on the pegs (information which you've learned so well, it's nearly impossible for you to lose). To begin, you could utilize your body parts to serve as pegs if you've got a list of things that you want to attach onto your nose, head and eyes, as well as your the limbs. You can also use this with everyday objects that you are confident that you will not forget. As you practice, it will become simpler for you brain keep ever more details thanks to the practice.

Pegging is a great way to use memories of the eye, you also make use of other senses like the smells and sounds to recall things. Like visual perception the senses of smell and sound are processed much faster by the brain. This is why that you cannot forget the scent of lavender in a matter of minutes. It's impossible to forget how you hear the sound of the piano. The ability to associate new information with these senses will help you keep the information permanently in your memory, instead of a unstable one. Try to recall the information through your senses. Next time you go to the grocery store, connect your shopping list to their scents, and you'll better chance of remembering everything.

Spatial awareness which refers to spatial and visual thinking is an essential ability. When driving and need to get between places and navigate through the busy streets. When you're trying planning an outdoor picnic that you plan, you engage in spatial thinking, making plans ahead, thinking about the way you would like everything to flow, the best way to reach your destination, the like. All of these activities require you to visualize as you plan, organize and arrange. But don't depend on your day-to-day actions to improve your spatial awareness because by performing the same tasks, your brain is in autopilot mode. That is, repeated actions don't increase your spatial awareness. To enhance your spatial abilities it is necessary to work on 3D mechanical games. Start by solving the classic Rubik's Cube. There are also visually-teasing puzzles. Other ways to learn include carpentry, pottery, or manipulating computer models in a 3D space. Simple tasks like making furniture using instructions can help you develop your spatial areas.

Video games are another great method to improve your visual awareness. Recent studies have demonstrated that playing video games can increase the ability to move and short-term memory. The games require players to focus across the screen in order to notice and react to the changing circumstances, thereby increasing your spatial awareness. Studies conducted in clinical settings have demonstrated how playing games stimulate previously inactive genes which are vital to build neural pathways that are necessary for spatial focus. Additional studies show the fact that video gaming could significantly increase your ability to pay attention.

Another option is to write down your dreams. If you happen to be thinking about something, try to remember the sequence of dreams. Take the time to write down every single detail as soon as you wake up. You'll realize that you're basically writing down your thoughts about the images you have in your mind They may not make sense but dreams are like they are. In this way, you can begin the process of creating. This is the type of practice that can increase the creativity of your brain. If you follow this strategy each time you think and write it down in words You will be able to enable your brain to become more imaginative and creative when it comes to nature.

To get your brain to concentrate effectively, you should practice meditative techniques. Begin by finding an empty space, then take a seat and concentrate on your breathing. Let your mind go completely. Avoid getting distracted by thoughts that are running through your mind. There will be times where you'll have thoughts whirling around your head however, try to concentrate only on breathing, and ignore all other thoughts. Try to shut out all background sounds. Then, consider the place you've been to. Imagine the way it looks and how the weather feels and then engage all your senses to focus on that specific location. Once you've reached that fully-engaged state, you'll realize that your brain has created a specific area using its stored memories and filling in the gaps by using its imagination. This will cause your brain to become more imaginative and creative over the course of.

Another excellent method to increase your creative abilities is playing the game of imaginary biography. It can be played by yourself or in a group with friends. The rules are easy Write down various words on pieces of paper that relate to fame, such as famous people landmarks, historical events or landmarks. Fold the paper in half and place them into an cap. Make a series of turns, and then pick one of the papers. Whatever word you find you must include it in your own personal biography about it over the following 30 minutes. This is a great method to exercise your brain. If you are struggling to create your own personal story with the most unimaginable factor Your brain will have to work harder to fill in the blanks by using its imagination and creative thinking.

Drawing with a pencil is another way to improve your brain. Research has proven that drawing with a pencil is among the most basic ways that children can demonstrate their creativity. When kids draw in the early years they may not be able to comprehend the concept at first, but as they get more practice, their doodles develop into useful drawings. Additionally, research has proven that drawing helps to arrange your thoughts, feelings and experiences. If you've ever had an issue with creativity it is possible to turn to drawing. It's a method for your brain to express itself in the way that is artistic when it is unable to respond with words. In order to develop your brain you can attempt to interpret drawings made by other people. If you are unable to think of something, then you can add to the sketches and continue adding until you've turned the sketch into something that is meaningful.

Thinking laterally is extremely important particularly when we wish to resolve a problem, but cannot find the solution. Lateral thinking is about having a new perspective rather than following the linear course when thinking creatively. We are prone to follow the path others have been following. We overuse logic and confine our own thinking within it. What happens? There is no solution to the problem. Because, digging a bigger than the original area won't alter the result but digging it in an another location could. This is a way is a good idea to improve your thinking laterally and expand your horizons. Ask yourself how many possible ways can you think of to connect the nine dots in an area using just 4 straight lines without removing your pen? Use a piece of paper to test various ways to connect them. This will help train your mind to think outside from the confines of. Try similar puzzles and exercises that require you to think outside of the box rather than following the trends.

The optical illusion is another efficient method to stimulate your brain. The optical illusions provide a glimpse into how the brain's creative process operates. The study of optical illusions and mental errors has shown that eyes don't actually see, but rather capture information that the brain can process. The brain associates the information it collects with the contextual context, analyzes it and processes it, then evaluates it. It's true that the ability to make sense of images is among the most imaginative actions our brains can perform. Optic illusions are regarded as excellent stimulators of creativity because they activate the right hemisphere of the brain (associated with creativity) and force your brain to view things in different ways in order to understand the picture. For exercise, explore different types of optical illusions, and try to interpret them.

The next item on the list next on the list is "Number workout". Like a workout at the gym can help you develop muscles, the number exercise stimulates your brain to improve the speed and intelligence. The exercise is a easy numerical exercise. It usually involves rapid fire arithmetic and simple maths problems such as subtractions subtraction, multiplication, and division. On first sight, the exercise may seem to be nothing extraordinary, however there's more to math exercises than what's apparent. Studies have proven that the nerve system of your brain has Axons, neurons and nerve fibers. All of these are involved in the transmission of signals to and from. The speed at which these signals are transmitted between your brain's neuron determines how quickly your brain processes information. You'll be amazed to learn that solving a simple math problem such as addition can increase the axons' insulation, that result in a greater speed of transmission of signals across neurons. In addition, research shows that mental arithmetic can improve in speed and accuracy. Moreover, more complex and intricate math problems such as trigonometry or algebra can boost your problem-solving capacity.

The problem is that we rely on calculators to perform these calculations However, you have to stimulate your brain to keep it sharp.

It is also possible to try a the visual math exercise to boost your intelligence. These workouts help your brain process information faster , which increases your intelligence. Also, if you have problems that would take some time to solve you'll be able to tackle it faster. It is possible to begin by solving simple geometric problems by using diagrams or tackle problems that require bar graphs and pie charts. These are great exercises that will strengthen your brain. When you are trying to solve math problems using visuals various parts of your brain are activated and are able to engage both the right and left hemispheres. You are able to comprehend the mathematical language using ways to understand the logical meaning. When solving math problems using visuals it can be difficult at first because a lot of information is given and you may be confused. However, with more details it will become more straightforward to solve a problem when compared to fewer details. Additionally, learning the diagrams of math problems could aid in solve the issue.

If you're looking to increase your thinking ability, Sudoku is your most effective option. In the past couple of years Sudoku became quite popular as a way to exercise your brain. It was first popularized in Japan in the late in the 1980s. But, it was originally named"the "Number Place" and the designer of the game was an American known as Howard Garns. It's a fun little game that has 9 squares arranged together to create a large square. Sudoku is essentially an exercise in logic. It is primarily based on numbers, but does not involve math. Engaging in Sudoku every day together with other puzzles and activities can help keep your brain engaged. Our brains age with time and gets worse due to the fact that our daily routine is usually linear. If we are doing things over and over the brain goes into its autopilot mode that isn't stimulating the brain as effectively. The game of Sudoku is a great way to provide a refreshing change to your routine, and will stimulate the brain and increase its ability to think rationally.

Riddles are brain-teasing games that aid your brain in enhance your critical thinking. Riddles can be an enjoyable method to involve your brain in training. They're closely related to logical fallacies which lead you to use incorrect logic. Because they are written in allegorical or metaphorical language they can be difficult to grasp initially. However, that's the essence of riddles. They're created to confuse you in order to make you think more deeply and focus your attention to figure out the right answer.

General intelligence is comprised of two parts of crystallized and fluid intelligence. It is the capability to discern meaning from chaos and discover solutions , while crystallized intelligence is the sum of all the information, knowledge and experiences you have accumulated throughout your lifetime. So, when kids are still young, they begin to learn languages more quickly, but as they grow older it is transformed into crystallized intelligence. It does not really stimulate your brain cells as much. However, if you begin to discover a new language as the adulthood, it will increase the activity of your brain since the process of learning a new language can be a challenging. It consumes many resources in your brain, but it can also strengthen your brain as a result. Clinical studies have proven that learning a language is among the most effective ways to guard your brain from the harms of the aging process. A study found that those who were bilingual experienced less mental decline in comparison to those who only spoke one language.

You never knew that you could become more proficient at reading comprehension and interpreting them! Actually reading comprehension can work your brain in a variety of ways. The ability to read and engage with the words that are used to help you comprehend works to improve your perception thinking, reasoning, problem solving and other cognition tasks. It is possible to begin by reading a few pages from books that contain comprehension exercises. Then, you will have to respond to the questions relating with the text. This method allows your brain to discern logical pitfalls from everyday situations. Your responses are generally the result of how well you interpret the meaning. In addition, it can activate you in your memory of visuals, your short-term memory, and speed with that your brain can transfer signals across the visual pathways.

Neuroplasticity experts have also pointed that training in music improves the brain's overall functioning and connectivity. A study from 1993 found that subjects performed better in the spatial reasoning test following listening to Mozart sonata. To help develop your brain you can either listen to music and learn how to play a new instrument. When you start playing an instrument that you have never played before your brain goes through major modifications. Research has shown an enormous increase in brain's speech perception, as well as the ability to discern emotions, and the ability to multitasking. The practice of playing music can force your brain to improve in solving problems in alternating tasks, and focusing. As brain development comes from the experiences that stimulate the brain and put a greater demands upon it. Hence, learning how to play an instrument that you can sing can be a powerful tool to create positive brain changes.

Chapter 11: Self Directed

Neuroplasticity

Now that you know that your brain is neuroplastic throughout the course of your life and you are able to use self-directed neuroplasticity to decide how you want your brain to work. For example, if are looking to improve your performance when it comes to social interaction, you can get your brain to become more comfortable performing in these scenarios and eventually change.

How does it work

The concept is that your brain functions through controlling your mind. If you did not have any kind of mind, then you'd be an automaton, and shouldn't be accountable for the crimes you commit... This is the feeling that you are not in a position of self-control. You are dependent on your brain.

Even if you don't recognize the fact that the brain controls your "mind" think about the higher order areas that govern those

118

of lower order to provide you with control. Higher order regions allow you to shift your focus and use your willpower to alter your behavior which in turn leads to changes in your brain (otherwise known as neuroplasticity).

The concept of self-directed neuroplasticity is based on:

*Attention

Everything can grab the attention of a person at any moment. This is an outcome of exposure to various types of stimuli. But, you have full control of the amount of focus you pay to an object or behavior, or even thought. It is possible to have a worrying thought that requires a lot of focus but you may choose to let it go and instead focus on something different. The goal is to concentrate on what you would like to accomplish to help lighten your brain and allow it to be wired to the way you would like it.

*Willpower (volition)

Attention is important however, it will do nothing to change the situation. You must go deep into the trenches to do some actual work. If you're trying to eliminate an unavoidable habit, such as compulsive behaviors, you need develop a strategy for redirect your attention to engage in another activity that will change the how your brain works. If you keep working the brain will begin firing up the brain circuits connected to the new task, in contrast to the unwelcome one.

*Brain activation

It happens because of an interaction between how you choose to manage your willpower and direct your focus. If you choose to concentrate on being grateful and feel happy the different area of the brain is likely to start to light up instead of being depressed. If you practice enough the part of your brain that is responsible for feeling grateful will be able to overcome the part that is that is associated with depression-related feelings, as you're making use of the brain more often.

*Consistency

The different brain regions are always competing to carry various tasks. The areas you use frequently will be more dominant than other regions. However the neural pathways and areas that you don't use as frequently are less likely to be affected or will slow down over time. The activities you perform every day are a huge influence in the performance of your brain, due in part to the way that neural networks you require to carry out these actions are strengthened over time, and those that are not used as often are weaker.

How do you use it?

I would like to think that you are aware that the substances you take and supplements, your sleep cycle and social groups, as well as your surroundings, and even your behavior all affect your brain's functioning. If you're conscious of the influences your brain has it is possible to alter them which could be doing more harm than positive effects. Here are some actions you can take to tap the ability of self-directed neuroplasticity

Awareness: Be aware of what you want to change. There are a myriad of things that you're aware of that you are not happy with, and other things you don't like in your life. Choose one at a time and be aware of the particular attitude, behavior or behavior that you'd like to alter.

Attention: Do not let your mind wander to another thing, instead pay full attention to creating an appropriate behavior or thought pattern. This requires lots of effort however, you must do your best. If you choose to focus on depression-related thoughts, the emotions will be magnified. In contrast If you choose to pay attention to gratitude, it increases the feeling of happiness.

*Volume: Remember that you'll be uncomfortable the first time you attempt to alter your brain. Everyone is wired differently and neuroplasticity process is designed to be effective, not a comfortable. Imagine being thrown into the swimming water pool and not knowing how to swim: the brain's choice to adapt or you drown. Although this may be slightly extreme, it is likely that you'll experience a level of resistance once you begin to make changes. But, if you keep your mind on gratitude and keep your determination and focus, your brain will change eventually.

Consistency: Be aware that your brain will have to adapt to new neural pathways that you introduce consistently. When the unwelcome thoughts occur, you should try connecting your newly formed neural networks for a minimum of 15 minutes. This shifts your attention on the negative thoughts and shift your focus to positive ones. This will eventually result in permanent changes to your brain as time passes. In time, the feelings of depression will disappear as your brain is buzzing with joy. To make changes, a consistent effort is essential.

*Brain changes: It's possible to alter the way your brain functions with concentrated effort. The changes to the brain are more firmly established with time. The longer you keep the habit that is healthy and the easier it is to keep it. This is why monks who practice kinds of meditation, such as mindfulness and compassion do not suffer from depression. Through years of training their brains are trained to feel positive emotions. However those who are always thinking about depressive thoughts will only strengthen the neural pathways that lead to depression.

The Importance of Doing The Right Choice Over Misguided Choices

Imagine you were applying the concept of self-directed plasticity to alter your brain's structure to master the new skill. Let's say tennis will be the new sport you would like to master. The question is how do you play it with enough skill to improve from being average proficient to becoming extremely proficient.

It is possible to buy an instrument and go about the park. It could be a good method to learn of the fundamentals, however it could be giving you the wrong information. It could teach your brain the wrong patterns of hitting the tennis ball the body's stance, footwork and the list goes on. It is important to remember that for you to obtain the results you desire, the best way to go is to partner with the top. If, for instance, you struggle with depression, it's best to seek out some or a few people who have succeeded in this and follow their advice rather than trying to lead yourself in a blind way.

If you're trying to feel less miserable you should probably try to seek assistance from someone who's had success in solving the issue instead of someone else who is struggling with the issue. Although their approach might not be the best for you, it is at least you're implementing a strategy that has proven to work, instead of trying to figure out the things you should be focusing your energy and focus on.

A broader view of self-directed brain plasticity

Though the intention is to help your brain to create new neural pathways and activated neurons It is recommended to take whatever action is needed. The power of attention and concentration can be very beneficial in forming neural pathways, however different methods and substances can help increase their effectiveness.

*Drugs: You might be tempted to try certain drugs and supplements to aid in changing a particular habit. It is crucial to make the changes in behavior while you are taking the drug to alter the way your brain functions. After you have withdrawn from the substance it is important to keep the behavior changes that encourage identical brain activities. It is possible to take an a specific substance from time to time to provide you with an early boost to change your behavior.

*Forced behavior: Forcing yourself to accept new behaviors can be a challenging job. A lot of people give up due to the uneasy emotions that accompany the degree of difficulties. Even though behavioral change is part of the process but you must also consider a mental perspective at the same time.

*Meditation: Meditation can aid in regaining your focus. Self-directed neuroplasticity is not able to be effective if you aren't in control of your focus. The more well-developed your focus is and the more you're not in the hands of the predominant neural patterns. There are many forms of meditation to produce specific changes to your brain's functioning.

Mindfulness: The practice of mindfulness will help you become more conscious of your thoughts and actions. It helps you be aware of your present mental state, and to refocus your focus whenever you're looking to change an unhealthy habit.

*Visualization: Visualization could result in changes to the brain, too. Research has shown that our subconscious doesn't be able to distinguish between actual and imagined things. Therefore when you imagine yourself playing an instrument or engaging in specific action, your brain believes it is an real-life incident. But, there are some who are unable to imagine accurately or precisely enough to trigger similar changes within the brain. However, the effectiveness of this technique is very significant and should not be overlooked.

It is it simple to master self-directed neuroplasticity?

It is all dependent on the particular behaviour you're trying to improve, how determined you are to make the changes and the level of change you'd like to see. Let's say, for instance, you're suffering from depression and you want to be satisfied, but aren't in a position to change your behavior. If you have set yourself up with a plan to boost your happiness, especially if you were depressed for many years it could take a while before you feel marginally better. This is due to the fact that changes in your brain is not something that happens over night. What can you do to learn to control your own neuroplasticity?

Passion: Your personal motivation or passion play an important role in determining the level of the difficulty involved in making the brain. The more eager you are to make a change and be more enthusiastic, the more inclined you'll be to work hard to conquer the hurdle.

Passion is the key to achieving results or remaining in the same place.

Make small adjustments If you're making significant changes in your daily routine it is possible that you will experience greater resistance than you normally. For instance, suppose you'd like to work at least an hour a day, but you haven't exercised in a while. Your brain might find the changes so dramatic that it feels "painful". You might find yourself coming up with reasons the reason you should stop or run out of energy, etc. It is because your brain was operating on neurons that were so powerful that it's going to require a significant period of time complete the switch. The only way to be successful is to make tiny changes.

Who could benefit?

Anyone can benefit if they comprehend and implement the concept of self-directed neuroplasticity. It's a reviving perspective that is backed by scientific research. The extent of your growth is contingent on the amount of exertion: pay focus and engage in different habits to aid your brain's adaptation to the new world. You'll likely feel uncomfortable throughout the process however, you'll eventually find a solution that will work. No matter if you're suffering from an injury to the brain, OCD, depression or anxiety disorders You can make your brain fire up and perform in the way you'd like it to.

Now that you understand the role of neuroplasticity and can power and is related will power are connected, how can you build the willpower of your brain.

Chapter 12: Techniques For Increasing Your Iq

This chapter you'll be taught proven, tested and well-established techniques to boost your intelligence. But , firstly, are aware that your intelligence can be determined through two variables? The majority of the time, only 50 percent of it is due to genetics. The remainder is up to the individual and how they can increase it. There are ways to boost your intelligence. Certain of them are discussed within this article.

IQ Enhancing Technique #1 Maintain the Sound Mind and Body

It is possible to boost your IQ by choosing to be aware of how to maintain your heart health. Every now and again you must make a conscious effort to increase the heartbeat. Also, sweating is an excellent idea when you want to fight memory loss. Things like running cycling, riding bikes or playing sports and swimming are beneficial in sharpening your mind. This assists in the delivery adequate oxygen into the brain. If you are doing this regularly and consistently, your brain's functions will improve and it will allow you to cope with stress well. In the end you will see that the IQ score will improve significantly.

IQ Boosting Technique #2: Write, Write, Write

If you're an author, you are extremely lucky. You are able to increase your brain's abilities every day. Do you remember the days when you were in school? You were prone to record every single thing. It is actually a beneficial practice as it increases your intelligence. It aids in learning because it aids in remembering the specifics of the writing you do.

If you're not a prolific writer You can still write frequently. Perhaps, you can keep a journal or a diary. This gives you an opportunity to write down every thought, idea and even every moment you'd like to recall. Don't stop noting them down. Every day you should try reading them over.

Reviewing them will aid you since it boosts the brain's capacity to retain information.

Did you realize that the most renowned geniuses of the past like Isaac Newton, Thomas Jefferson as well as Albert Einstein all have journals? In addition, they were thought to be writers who were obsessed with their journals. Perhaps this will motivate the reader to write one.

IQ Enhancing Technique #3 to avoid boredom by every methods

Couch-sitting an indication of boredom. It is therefore recommended to stop the habit of watching TV too often. Mom was right in her advice that television can cause you to be dumb.

Instead of sifting through your television channels or sitting in a slumber on your sofa Why not try the crossword puzzle? If you own an chess set, you can try taking on yourself. Increase your logical skills through keeping your hands busy and not succumbing to the lure of boredom.

Technique for boosting IQ #4: Purchase the Rubik's Cube

If the barbells represent muscles Rubik's Cube is to the brain. We should be grateful to the person who designed the cube in 1974. In 1974, a year that was defining that was in Hungary, Erno Rubik was capable of creating an item that helped many people smarter. The Rubik's Cube can increase your ability to use geometry and visualizing 3D images. Keep your mind occupied because the Rubik's Cube presents you a new problem that needs that needs to be solved each time!

Enhancing IQ Technique #5: Accept the pleasure of being a lifetime student

You must be ready to learn something new each day throughout your life. Learning doesn't stop after the school. However, the majority of neural pathways developed were formed as you reached school years. To sustain your growth, you must constantly look for new knowledge.

Everyday, you must take a chance to try something that is new. If you can, enroll in a class. In the following years, you could be interested in registering at The

Graduate School. This will allow you to expand the boundaries of your mind.

Chapter 13: The Foods That Help

You Become More Educated

Healthy eating as well as eating healthy food can boost your brain's power. Certain foods can enhance the brain's capabilities and aid it function effectively. It is essential to take in foods that are brimming of antioxidants, fibre, and omega-3 fats. Here are a few "smart food items" included in your food routine:

Avocado It's a fruit that contains monounsaturated fats which can aid in allowing the blood flow better and lower blood pressure. Additionally, it contains Vitamin E.

Blueberries are often referred to as brainberries since they are thought to be the most nutritious food to nourish the brain. They shield your brain against stress, and also reduce the risk of developing Alzheimer's or dementia. They're high in fiber and can help maintain a healthy blood sugar. Drinking a cup of blueberries a day whether frozen or fresh will increase your brain's capabilities.

Nuts - A one ounce of nuts daily can immediately improve your energy levels because of the complex carbohydrates they contain. They also have vitamin E that aids in the cognitive functions that the brain performs. Some good nuts to boost your brain power are hazelnuts, walnuts, cashew nuts Brazil nuts, almonds , and filberts. You can also make use of almond butter and peanut butter. Do not use nuts that contain seasonings or sweeteners and salted nuts.

Seeds contain beneficial fats Vitamin E as well as protein, antioxidants and magnesium. Magnesium, a mineral, helps boost the energy levels in the brain. The most suggested seeds include flax seeds, sesame seeds, sunflower seeds, and Tahini.

Wild salmon - It is rich in many omega-3 that are essential for the development of your brain. Omega 3 are fats known to improve the brain's alertness and improve memory. They also boost your mood, decrease the risk of developing dementia-related diseases, aids in preventing depression, anxiety, and hyperacidity. Other fishes with omega-3 include sardines and herring.

Beans beans Lentils along with black beans supply a constant glucose levels and your brain requires glucose in order to function. The glucose in the beans acts as fuel, therefore it is recommended to consume half a cup of beans each day.

Oatmeal is loaded with fiber and can keep you going throughout the first part of the day. They are great for heart health and turn help keep the brain healthy.

Coffeeis great for your brain as it is a source of fiber that benefits the cardiovascular system. It also acts as an instant energy boost, increases the range of your attention and boosts your ability to react. A study has also been conducted which shows that coffee drinkers reduce the risk of developing Alzheimer's diseases by 30 percent. The recommended amount is 2 to 4 cups per day but no more than that.

Tea contains catechines, which is a potent type of antioxidant that improves circulation of blood through the body. It also aids in focusing and stay focused on your task. It should be brewed, not powdered or stored.

Dark chocolate-Chocolate that has 70 percent cocoa is the ideal type for your brain as it's packed with flavonoids and natural stimulants such as caffeine, and aids in release endorphins, which enhance mood. Every day, at minimum 12 ounce of chocolate can bring the above benefits, plus being aware that it could help reduce blood pressure.

Pomegranate- This fruit is loaded with antioxidants that shield your brain from the negative effects on free radicals. It is also possible to take a taste of the juice if don't like drinking raw fruit.

Oysters are high in essential nutrients to a healthy brain, such as selenium, magnesium and protein.

Garlic Fresh garlic is superior since it decreases the amount of cholesterol known as bad cholesterol and strengthens your cardiovascular system. Garlic protects your brain through the high levels of antioxidants.

Eggs are a super foods that contain selenium, which can boost your mood. They are rich in protein and fat that help to sustain the energy levels of your brain for a long periods of time. The yolk of an egg contains Choline, which is a memory enhancement nutrients. Choline is the primary ingredient of two brain cells- the phosphatidylcholine, and the aphingomyel.

Tomatoes are rich in lycopene an antioxidant known to stop the development of dementia.

Leafy green vegetables - They are well-known for their iron-rich content which can benefit the brain. The lack of iron can lead to fogged thinking, low moods and fatigue. Therefore, eating vegetables can prevent these issues.

Drinking waterThe ability to keep your brain well-hydrated by drinking at minimum 8 glasses of fluids every day is essential to help your brain perform at its highest level. According to experts in health that dehydration is the main reason for memory loss, so to prevent it from happening ensure that you remain completely hydrated all day long.

Kelp Kelp Kelp is a variety of seaweed that is rich in Iodine, magnesium and calcium. The most important nutrients essential to develop and grow the brain is the iodine. Iodine deficiency is among the main causes of stunted growth and issues with learning in children. It also can cause mental impairment.

Cacao is rich in levels of antioxidants and epicatechin compounds that can stimulate the brain specifically its memory and learning faculties. Keep your mind sharp by drinking a the delicious hot cacao drinks or a cooling, refreshing smoothies of cacao.

Beets are a rich source of Vitamin B which helps the brain process information and information quickly. They also have antidepressants.

Chapter 14: The Way to Build An

Iron Trap Memory

A brief description of memory

Coding is the first stage in creating an entirely new memory. It allows the object that is of interest to be converted into a structure which is then capable of being kept in your brain. Then , it can be remembered in the future from the long-term or short-term memory.

There are four kinds of encryption.

Acoustic Encoding

The memory holds sound, such as the sounds we hear and words. They're stored for future use and later recovered. This is basically the kind of memory can be used to recall conversations or hearing our parents calling us by name when we were an infant.

Visual Encoding

That's the place we save the sensory and visual information. It's stored temporarily in the iconic memory, before being stored for the long term. The amygdala plays an essential role in this process as it is able to accept visual input as well as the input of our emotion system, too. Thus, our memories of visuals are correlated with either negative or positive values.

Tactile Encoding

It is the way that something feels real through our senses of contact. The physical body of ours respond to the touch of objects and then that memory is put in our memory for the long term.

Semantic Coding

Semantic encoding actually describes what you feel emotionally when you think about a moment. Imagine the first time your child was wrapped their fingers around yours, or recalling the first moment you lost a loved pet or family member. The semantic encoding of our memories is a way to store and preserve the essence of our emotions.

It is generally accepted that short-term memory encode is typically created through audio encoding, while memories for the long term are created through semantic encoded. It is believed that sleeping aids in the retention of memories and has been confirmed by numerous research studies. Additionally that, the more often a particular memory is replayed and repeated and re-played, greater the likelihood that it is to remain in memory. A notable exception to this is when you remember something deeply because the meaning-encoding that occurred was deep and lasting.

Strategies to Enhance Memory

There are a variety of methods you can employ to increase your memory. These techniques are all focused upon improving overall health as well as developing your brain.

Make sure you get enough exercise and sleep

As mentioned, exercise increases the flow of oxygen into your brain. This can help it to function more efficiently. It can also aid in the production of the brain's chemicals and safeguard the brain cells. If you're deficient in sleep the brain can't continue to function as it should. Additionally, the time we sleep , our brains go through the data from our day and decides what is essential and what needs to be removed.

Enjoy and be social

Research has proven that having an open and meaningful connection with loved ones and friends can be a great boost to our mental health as well as keeping our brains healthy. There was no reason for us to live in a solitary environment. A study conducted by Harvard found that people who lead the most active interactions with others are much less likely experience a decline in memory.

Furthermore laughing is good to your brain. It not only stimulates your brain's emotional part, but it stimulates every part within your brain. Laughter is the most effective treatment.

There is a lot of laughter within your own life through sharing humorous personal stories, moving towards laughter and sharing the moment by engaging with people who are positive and surrounded by the reminders to laugh, such as posters or toys and paying attention to your children. Kids are masters in letting their lives go and having fun.

Do away with Stress

The brain is the most dangerous enemy , and it can lead to chronic stress that causes brain damage and destruction of the hippocampus. The hippocampus is crucial for making new memories as well as recollecting memories from the past. Try some meditation techniques or mindfulness to get rid of stress. Find an expert if nothing you do can help.

Eat Well

Your brain requires fuel, just like your body. If you're feeding it wrong foods, it will not function as effectively as it ought to. Therefore, you should consume not only a well-balanced diet, but also an optimum diet for your brain.

Increase your intake of omega-3 by eating more walnuts, fish as well as flaxseed, kidney beans and pumpkin seeds and broccoli.

Reduce your intake of calories and saturated fats , such like red meats, milk in whole form butter, cheese Ice cream, red meat, and cream. Studies have proven that an increased risk of developing dementia and diminished concentration is related to increased consumption of saturated fats and calories.

Eat your vegetables and fruits and fruits, not just because your mother advised you to and so on, but because they're brimming with antioxidants, which protect your brain cells from being damaged. They weren't wrong when she advised you to take more fruit and vegetables. Consider eating more blueberries, cantaloupe, apricots, and bananas as a way to get started.

Consume more green tea as it is a rich source of polyphenols, which combat free radicals that could damage the brain cells. Green tea consumption regularly has been proven to boost the alertness and memory of people.

Drink grape juice or wine in moderation. Limit yourself to one glass per woman and two for males, since small quantities have been proven to boost memory and cognitive function. However, more than that will cause brain cells to die.

Exercise Your Brain

When you're an adult your brain has developed thousands of neuronal pathways to process information and locate it quickly and efficiently solve common issues. But if you adhere to the well-established paths and do not change them from them, your brain will get inactive. This is why you should select brain exercises or simply enjoy something different. There are three essentials to an exercise for the brain.

It's important to ensure that it's something completely that's completely new. The thing you decide to do should be something completely new and outside of your comfort zone to be effective.

It should be difficult. If you find it to be not challenging, it's probably not something new to you or is it? It's similar to learning a new instrument or language or perhaps completing an online crossword.

It should be something that is enjoyable. The more engaged you are in a particular sport the more likely you'll be able to recall it.

Make use of Mnemonic Devices

As was explained previously the term "mnemonic device" refers to an item that you have come across with something that you would like to keep in mind. There are many different methods, however they all follow the same basic idea. The other fundamentals are:

Visualizing your image: Your image should represent positive and pleasant, and colorful and exaggerated. This can help you remember it more easily.

Acrostic: It is a sentence in which the first letter in every word signifies something you want to keep in mind. For instance the treble clef EGBDF can be remembered by saying 'every good boy is perfectly.'

Acronym: It's an expression that is created by taking the initial letters of the keyword or concepts and making a new word. For instance "HOMES" is the name of the great lake system (Huron, Ontario, Michigan, Erie, and Superior).

There are a variety of other methods available. You must find the one that works for you and continue to use it. We'll now move to the subject of habits and their role on your brain.

Chapter 15: Spiritually

This chapter might not be so easy to accept as a fact since in our current time humans have reduced our knowledge of life to only five senses. If the experience isn't compatible with our five senses the information that has been presented to us is rejected. But, that isn't the case.

Whatever your background or your current culture or religion, humans have experienced more of this sixth sense of the spiritual world more than we'd like to admit. For centuries, we believed in the gods of our times however it was different with time. This is a simple fact: we're not mere physical beings. our souls are divine beings.

There is more to us than what we can see in our mirrors and encounter in our lives. We all have certain thoughts about people, events or situations that are difficult to describe. This suggests the fact that humans are also spiritual. There's even a remarkable study which showed that children were born with an inclination to believe in the supernatural as well as an over-powering god over naturalism.

It is quite surprising that our brains are able to respond positively to acts of spirituality. Things we do to assist in the development of our spirituality are also beneficial to the development and well-being of our brains. It's as if our brains connect with the reality the fact that our souls are divine beings.

I hope that after you read this chapter, you'll agree that you are more than an individual. You would realize that you are much more than what you see in the mirror. There exists more that the eyes of the natural.

Meditation and Prayer

Two elements that every religion is able to do in a way these are the practices of prayer and meditation. It is important to consider isn't the shared characteristics across all the religions of the world in relation to this type of practice, however rather the numerous benefits and effects they can bring to your brain when practiced regularly over time. Simply put, putting your time in the growth of these practices will not only increase your appreciation for these practices, but also increase the performance and capacity the brain.

While many people believe that religion and science are in conflict in some areas however, there's something they are both on the same page the fact that prayer and meditation can transform the way a person lives their life. The most appealing aspect is that the results don't discriminate just towards the same people group social class, socioeconomic status, or geographical location. It is able to everyone who decides to follow these fundamental techniques.

Through a variety of research studies We have discovered some of the numerous benefits these practices can bring to users. One benefit that the practice of meditation and prayer produce is the actual expansion in the grey matter within our brains. If you are able to take time in alone time to meditate the brain will expand and increase the amount of energy it uses in the brain region which is responsible for focus and concentration.

Through meditation and prayer it is possible to find it easier to relax your mind. The areas that are responsible for soothing you in fighting, flee or freeze response will grow and be able to help you remain calm during stressful times. It won't be as hard to stay into control of your thoughts and rapid breathing like it was previously.

If you decide to sit for 15 minutes of meditation when you are struggling with writing block, it can help you to be more imaginative. You'll feel a higher feeling of enthusiasm for taking on the project before you, particularly if you meditated to imagine your accomplishments and your life in the future. The effectiveness of prayer and meditation has been exposed to the world by science as revolutionary that doctors, CEO's entrepreneurs, doctors and others are seeing it as a necessity to achieve the success of their business.

If you're thinking about how you can start or how to start, I would suggest you to choose an hour when you can are able to take 15 minutes to reflect or pray during one day. When you've completed one day, I'd like you to decide to continue for four consecutive days simultaneously. Why do you need to wait four days? Because it only takes four days of doing these tasks to get your brain started developing the new pathways for neural development. Your brain will transform its chemical makeup because you decided to keep doing this in four days!

That's it If you decide to let your brain be the main focus of the spiritual realm, you'll discover it much easier to be a meditative and prayer. The result of spending the time to meditate for 15 minutes every day will assist your brain in physical expand, you'll be able to manage stress in a more healthy way, and increase your creativity. What a simple act you can do to live the beauty we're meant to experience!

Chapter 16: Nutrition and Supplementation to Increase Brain Power

Overall, the negatives could outweigh the advantages in the case of using nootropics to increase or reduce the quantity of specific neurotransmitters.

But that's not to suggest there's not a method to boost the power of your brain with some outside help. The trick is to focus on the long-term health of your brain instead of attempting to gain an immediate boost in your cognitive abilities.

This is easy when you follow the proper diet. Diet is essential to brain health , and most of us aren't aware how important it is in this area.

Let's look at the various nutrients and supplements can be used to boost the power of your brain...

Amino Acids

Amino acids are the primary building components of protein. If you consume any kind of meat the brain breaks it down into amino acids, and then recombine them to create tissues in your body. These tissues can be used by the brain, so eating more amino acids could be utilized to increase the body's ability to grow and repair the brain!

However, this isn't the point at which the significance of amino acids stops. The amino acids are also vital for the production of a variety of neurotransmitters. For instance, ltyrosine is used to make dopamine while tryptophan (discussed earlier) is the main ingredient in creating serotonin. Some, such as l'theanine, can directly affect the brain, and in this case , it's an euphoric effect. L-carnitine can boost energy on the brain, by improving the efficiency of the mitochondria (more on this in a moment!).

We've seen this with 5-HTP it's possible to consume a lot in these amino acids by themselves and cause immediate changes in the amounts of neurotransmitters. However, this causes problems as we've observed and, contrary to popular belief that this isn't an advantage.

Therefore, the best option is to concentrate on creating an appropriate mix of as many amino acids as you can. Simply eating a lot of protein or supplementing with amino acids products, it is possible to supply the brain with all the ingredients it requires to produce all of the neurotransmitters it needs whenever it requires these. This makes it more efficient in achieving every mental state, ensuring that you have the ability to maximize your concentration, focus and memory all simultaneously.

The easiest way to gain a large amount of amino acids? Consume plenty of eggs. Eggs are among the few complete proteins, in that they are a complete source essential amino acids the brain can't make by itself. Additionally they also contain Choline which is the precursor of excitatory neurotransmitter Acetylcholine. They're an excellent source for healthy saturated fats too, and since the brain is made primarily out of oil, that's an extremely vital and beneficial element.

Vitamins and Minerals

It's the same for numerous minerals and vitamins. They also help make a variety of neurotransmitters which are so desired by those who want to improve their efficiency and focus.

Vitamin B6 specifically can be used to produce numerous neurotransmitters. Vitamin C is likewise essential to increasing serotonin levels and boost the mood, as well as protecting against diseases (which is accompanied by the neurotransmitter cytokines, which is an inhibitory one).

There are plenty of different roles for minerals and vitamins too. Vitamin B12 and iron B12 both assist in blood flow through the production of greater red blood cells. Vitamin D aids in controlling hormones and specifically testosterone. Zinc plays an important role in the development of neuroplasticity. Magnesium is also a powerful ally in fighting anxiety and depression.

In short, if don't get the micronutrients you require and require, then you're not giving your brain the nutrients it requires to function properly.

That's why it is important to stay away from processed food items. Anything that's very artificial, like an Mars Bar, bag of crisps or McDonald's hamburger will have calories that will fill you up but they won't provide the essential nutrients needed to be able to function. It's possible to live, but you'll be tired slow, unfocused and less productive in the end.

Consume healthy smoothies, salads as well as plenty of fruits and vegetables, and you'll see that you feel healthier and more alert. The best option is a multivitamin, and if you choose the correct one, it's a great way to boost the performance of your brain and overall health and wellbeing.

Vasodilators

If you're seeking an immediate boost to your brain that can be obtained from food and supplements that are safe and foods, look for vasodilators. A vasodilator can be defined as any substance that dilates blood vessels (veins and the arteries). This allows more blood and oxygen to circulate around your body, which results in more oxygen reaching your brain.

One of the most popular among those who love nootropics vinpocetine is because it targets the brain specifically as well as the prefrontal cortex more specifically. This means you're receiving more energy to the region of the brain responsible for problem-solving and planning and some have described the sensation as "a cool bath for the brain'.

Cognitive Metabolic Enhancers

This is a fancy name for anything that boosts the brain's energy levels, and typically, this refers to things that boost the effectiveness of mitochondria. Mitochondria are the energy-producing cells of your cells. They are floating in the cytoplasm, and make use of ATP and glucose to fuel your body's functions, including your brain function!

Numerous factors can aid your mitochondria function better, and include

CoQ10 and lutein, as well as l-carnitine PQQ, and more. This is the combination of amino acids as well as minerals, vitamins and other lesser-known nutrients that are found in supplements.

Another option is to simply eat well-balanced and healthy diet. However, you can boost your energy levels with creatine. Creatine is an ingredient that is often utilized by bodybuilders and athletes. Its main purpose is to convert the used ATP (adenosine as well as ADP) to usable ATP. Also, it recycles adenosine, which gives you extra energy for your workout.

The latest surprise is that it also enhances brain function by increasing the efficiency of energy for brain cells. It helps the brain recycle its ATP also, meaning you'll get a minute or two of additional energy when you are working at your maximum. Research shows that those who use creatine experience an additional boost in their IQ and this is certainly a highly efficient nootropic that has no risk of side effects or dangers!

Creatine is made naturally by the liver, and it can be obtained through your diet (sources like beef). But, the most effective way to experience a significant increase is to utilize it as a supplement - search to buy creatine monohydrate.

Omega 3 Fatty Acid

Omega 3 fatty acids are an excellent antioxidant discovered in tuna, as well as other fish that are oily along with several nuts and other sources. What is what makes omega 3 beneficial for the brain is that it improves 'cell membrane permeability'. This means that it makes the walls of cells of neurons slightly more permeable and allows things to move through a less easily. This includes neurotransmitters and nutrients and much more. In other words, it basically makes neurons more responsive and provides a little increase in your energy levels.

Antioxidants

Antioxidants are crucial to looking after your brain's health. This includes Vitamin C, Omega 3 Resveratrol, and a myriad of other micronutrients.

In essence, antioxidants function by neutralizing free radicals which are substances that harm cells when they come in contact with them. They could even cause cancer if they travel through the nucleus, causing DNA damage!

Consuming antioxidants is an extremely important aspect of your overall health. They can help lower the risk of getting sick through strengthening your immunity. But what we're most currently interested in is how this could boost the power of your brain over time by preventing brain cells from harm and possibly lowering the chance of developing tumors later on in your life.

Chapter 17: Eliminate Negative Influences

This is likely to be one of the most difficult chapters, and I've been waiting to write about it to this point, since I don't want you to be overwhelmed. A little bit of momentum prior to getting to this point can aid in gaining clarity, after you've taken a step back, analyzed your thoughts and made the effort to change them by adopting healthier, more effective ways of living.

Eliminating the negative influence from your existence covers lots of space, which is filled with different elements depending on the individual. Influences that are negative do not appear like everyone else It is essential not to be too involved in comparisons with other people. Nobody is superior to you simply because they're not struggling in like you struggle. I can assure you that all those who seem to live life in a perfect way on social media are dealing with their own challenges. As we've done in the previous chapters, now it's time to concentrate on yourself and eliminate the distractions that are holding you backor, even more that are forcing you to go forward.

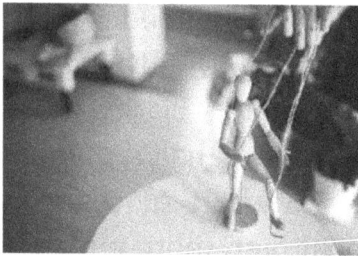

Get out the list you made from a few years ago, that lists all the causes and reasons for overthinking within your own life. There are likely to be events that occurred to you in the past and persist around, or previous traumas, or poor treatment received from other people. Perhaps you've written down events such as a boss who isn't a good one in the workplace, or a a pal who keeps trying to persuade you to be a sexy in her presence, or video clips on your social media feeds which show images of what you're supposed be, and you're feeling unhappy. Once we've made one step forward in our journey to transform the habit of thinking too much into focused achievement It's time to take a examine your personal life and figure out the extent to which negative influences are still in place. It's possible that you've eliminated significant sources of stress or stress and negative emotions however are there handful of them still within your life that are hindering you from achieving your goals? Each person's list will be completely different. I'm certainly not trying to substitute for the services of counselors. However, with a clearer head you'll be able recognize that certain influences are causing damage rather than positive effects. It's up to you to take action in these areas, however I'm able to offer a bit of help on the way.

First off, it's difficult to cut the ties to someone or something who's been happy within your life for a long period of time, even if the presence is ultimately detrimental. Many times people only see

167

only what they would like to see and steer clear of anything that could be challenging. This is probably what you were at first when you first realized it was the right time to change your ways.

The removal of any negative influence that are affecting your life is crucial to your growth. It's very easy to start such a path and succeed only to slide backwards due to the negative influences you allowed to influence your life and again. Be confident however, it's important not to undervalue the power of people or influences in your life. Even the most knowledgeable of us have been fooled by time to time in the form of fraud in the form of a marketing campaign or a lie told by an individual we believe in. If you have someone you know who is causing a negative impression upon you, it might be time to start a serious discussion.

Chatting with friends

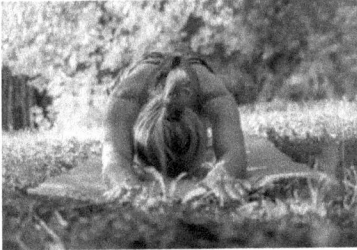

Let's first discuss how to interact with acquaintances. In the course of a good friendship we are taught to ignore the little details about the person's personality , or their character which we don't think are ideal. No one is perfect, but your friendship is more significant than the majority of the little flaws. There may have been disputes and arguments that were not so great and if your relationship is strong enough to endure these events circumstances, you'll be aware that the bond you share with your partner is solid. However, sometimes the things we ignore can actually be a lot more than we imagine them to be , and they need to be dealt with.

There are numerous kinds and types of harmful influences which could be sparked by the perspective of a friend. Your task is to decide whether these influences are hindering your progress towards becoming a happierand more productive person. If you can answer yes, no matter how difficult it is accepting, then it could be time to discuss with your partner about getting rid of the influence or perhaps cutting off all ties.

This is not an easy choice to make, and it can be difficult initially. However, if you take plenty of time to reflect on the situation and then keep returning to the same hard reality it is definitely an excellent idea to get away from this influence.

Make sure not to have the conversation become confrontational. Even if the conversation turns to be a struggle the best approach to tackle it is from the perspective of how much you appreciate the time you spent with your companion.

Begin by sitting down and discussing the subject by thoroughly explaining what you're doing to improve your life. Tell them that you're making a number of challenging adjustments to lead an active, healthy life. Tell the story of how you've been struggling with the same mentality for years without success and now it's time to get rid of the influences that hinder you from achieving your goals.

The issue may not be so grave that you need to break off all ties to your friend. It could be an issue that you must request your friend to stop talking about around you. If they are known to talk all the time and criticize others, and you notice that this is fueling your thoughts of obsessive thinking and overthinking, inform your friend that you're not going to talk about these things with them any longer.

It could be due to drug addiction or alcohol abuse or another negative influence that your friend is taking over you. In either of these cases the person who truly cares about you and your well-being will accept when approached with integrity and honesty position. Don't accuse the person who is damaging you. They may think their way of life is working for them and they aren't planning to stop. But that doesn't mean that they aren't willing to alter their behaviors around you to help you achieve your goals.

Consider a different option. It is possible to start talking with your friends or family members about the things you're trying to accomplish in your life. They might be excited at the thought of doing the same thing for themselves. By having a candid discussion with your close friends and family, you could gain an ally and a partner to follow this road towards greater clarity. Do not be afraid to speak with your friends from a position of vulnerability and honesty. It could prove to be a significant and positive influence in the lives of others!

Chatting with a friend or a partner

Discussing with a friend what they could be doing to negatively impacting you in a way is difficult however, talking to your family member or partner is likely be a lot more difficult. If you're lucky enough to have positive, positive influencers in your life, consider yourself extremely fortunate. If you're experiencing a relationship that is toxic to some degree it is vital to resolve the issue in the earliest time possible. While making the issue on whether or not you should end a relationship with someone you love but it is crucial not to misinterpret issues that can be resolved by discussion and dialogue with issues that aren't. Everything must start with honest and clear communication. Research has shown that a substantial portion of marriage problems result from poor communication. Incorrect communication can transform a miscommunication into something painfully hurtful. If something you or a loved one said or did hurt you, it could be that it was a mistake from their side. It's not the scenario for everyone, however, when you've had a positive and supportive relationship with the loved one, there's a greater possibility that the issue is that is as easy to fix as the miscommunication.

If, however, you've been through an extensive history of abuse of one kind or another, it's time to build the support you need and take on the negative effects directly. Do not disappear without a discussion unless the situation you're in could put you in danger physically. If that's the case, it's essential to leave the scene immediately.

However, if it's the case to break up your boyfriend or chatting with your spouse or family member regarding how you can break certain bad habits that are affecting you, the best way to go is to reserve the time to have a serious discussions. It is essential that you do not begin the discussion by becoming confrontational. Be open and give some background and explanations of why you are required to discuss. Disturbing your loved one will not assist you.

In the event that you have to speak with a person sincerity and openness are the best ways to go. Don't be the sole one talking and give your loved one or friend an opportunity to talk to them and express how feels. If your relationship has redeeming characteristics and is worthy of taking care of, then you'll be able to reach an agreement and understanding to move forward.

Allow yourself some time following breaking up or cutting off the ties

If your choice was to cut off the negative influences that have impacted the world, it is important to allow yourself time to recuperate and move through your feelings. Don't attempt to go back to where you started If you're struggling and require time to grieve the loss. It's normal, even if the thing you've gotten rid of affected you negatively. Humans have a tendency to become habitual and if a routine is abruptly removed out of our daily lives, you're bound be feeling the effects when we adjust. You might need a few days or two, or perhaps some weeks, or perhaps a whole month. This is fine. If you're at your best, return to review your goals, and continue moving ahead.

The most dangerous thing you can do is to try to soothe your feelings with a rebound. Nothing is more harmful to yourself or someone else than relying on another person and their emotional bond to ease your own feelings. Although it may be attractive, it's essential to take care of yourself and locate better ways to get through the loss you feel after a breakup. Rely on the people in your life who be there for you and love you. Don't be afraid to ask for help from a stranger.

Other negative influences

After we've dealt with some of the most difficult subjects Let's discuss some other negative influences that could have to be dealt with in your daily life.

We touched on healthy eating habits in the chapter on healthy habits. Food habits that are unhealthy are among of the toughest ways to get rid of because they're so instantly satisfying. This is also true with other addictions like alcohol and drugs. Both provide immediate feelings of excitement and joy. Do not let guilt enter into play when you look at your eating routines. Everyone has issues with eating healthy and the fact that you are unable to resist eating that chocolate bar at your workplace vending machine each day does not make you weak or a weak person. Recognizing that it's a bad habit is a good place to begin.

It's time to take small steps. Do not decide in the future, after having consumed chocolate every single throughout the last two years, that you're going to never eat chocolate ever again. I'm telling you...it won't happen.

Limit your consumption of chocolate to one each week. That's right. If you eat the Twix bar or some other item everyday, select one day of the week to make a commitment to not eating chocolate on that day. It's easy to begin making positive changes to your diet. While this chapter is about eliminating the negative influences completely however, it is important to remember that changing our behavior and removing unhealthy habits is not something that can be done in a single day.

If you purchase your chocolate from the same spot every single day, there are ways to stop this habit. Take a different route from your desk and, even if it's longer, and that doesn't go through the vending machine, the snack counter or cafeteria in the workplace. Naturally, this can be adapted to the environment you are in, but being in a location that has chocolate can have a negative impact on your behaviour because the place signals to your brain the idea that it's the right time to indulge in chocolate.

The same concept applies to advertisements. If you've seen those pictures of juicy hamburgers on commercials on television It's not that they're trying show their product, but they are also subconsciously informing your appetite and creating an impression to your brain that equates hunger and craving hamburgers every time you watch the commercial.

To eliminate this negative effect Try to minimize your exposure to these advertisements. It might be difficult since these ads are all over the place. However, with a bit of imagination I'm certain you'll discover ways to eliminate the influence of these ads out of your everyday routine.

As we've previously discussed that a large portion of negative influence comes from television and images we see in them that affect our emotional state as we associate positive aspects with the advertisements that we see each day. To remove all the influence you can will do great things for your self-esteem and positive outlook. All you need is one tiny change each day.

In the supermarket instead of looking at the perfect bodies and magazines on the covers try listening to the conversations that surround you. You might even start conversations with a person in the queue, like we've discussed earlier. This will help break the habit of looking at an image and instantly looking at yourself in relation to the image you are seeing.

The same influence is present on smartphones as well as other devices. It's not easy to stay clear of these ads, however, a good place to start is to check all your feeds from social networks and cease following people who promote nutrition or fitness products. You should make sure you block ads that are constantly appearing on your feeds that you don't want be seeing any more. Also the most effective way to get rid of this negative influence from your life is be to reduce the time you spend on your mobile generally. Replace the time you use the internet for with something that is more healthy for your mind such as something on your list of hobbies and practices to implement to your daily routine. It might be difficult initially, like breaking every bad habit is always difficult however, you'll soon begin to feel and see the positive impact in clearing your mind of the negative factors.

Another influence that can be negative is difficult to identify initially, since they can appear as beneficial and essential to personal improvement. If you're prone to listening to others around you and seeking their opinions, it could be time to remove that dependence to become more independent in your thinking process and habit formation. Just like I said nobody is more knowledgeable than you do. And the fact that something works for someone else, it doesn't necessarily mean it's going to perform also. Therefore, put down the Dr. Phil and get out your notebook. Pay attention to your mind and your body. It's going to be much simpler now that you've accomplished many things to help you find your path to becoming a more fulfilled you. Be proud that you've performed the entire lifting for yourself!

Change your career or job circumstance

In the world of negative influence, nothing could be more dangerous than the gradual, slow death of a dead-end job. If you graduated from high school or college with huge goals and ideas for your future, only to have them vanish after you accepted an uninteresting but steady job with a company you're not even interested in It could be draining your life of every motivation, excitement and energy.

If you're in this situation are in this situation, you're not alone. The current society encourages and even lauds those who are willing to put their bodies to earn an income. We're bombarded with messages from an early age that success means money and accountability. However, as we've considered the more you accumulate the more clutter you create in your home and mind as well as the stress that you add to your daily life.

Life isn't all about gain. As we've discussed in the previous article on minimalist living, fulfillment doesn't come from having belongings or climbing up a ladder in your career. If the profession isn't something you enjoy or are enthusiastic about, it's probably not worth the time and commitment. It's too short to do that.

It could be the last and largest obstacle between you and the person you want to be. As we approach the conclusion of this text and your new affirmation as a reenergized human having a clear and positive mind and a body that is full of positive influence and knowledge, be sure that the place in which you'll be spending most of your time during the year is one that you really want to be. Do not do this or go after this because others suggest it's the right choice. Do it because that's what you'd like to be.

Conclusion

I am very excited to relay this knowledge to you. I am extremely happy to have learned and are able to implement these methods in the future.

I hope that this book was useful in helping you understand the brain's changes and how you can utilize it to fulfill your goals.

It is now time to begin by using this information to hopefully lead a healthier and more fulfilled life!

Don't be one of those who simply reads this book and does not apply it. the techniques included in this book will only be beneficial if you apply the strategies!

If you know anyone else who might benefit from the advice provided here , please tell them about this book.

Thank you for your kind words and good luck!